# the**facts**

# Epilepsy in women

also available in the**facts** series

# thefacts

# Epilepsy in women

## TIM BETTS

Retired. Previously Reader in Neuropsychiatry
University of Birmingham
UK

## HARRIET CLARKE

Primary Teacher
UK

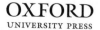
OXFORD
UNIVERSITY PRESS

# OXFORD
UNIVERSITY PRESS

Great Clarendon Street, Oxford OX2 6DP

Oxford University Press is a department of the University of Oxford.
It furthers the University's objective of excellence in research, scholarship,
and education by publishing worldwide in

Oxford  New York

Auckland  Cape Town  Dar es Salaam  Hong Kong  Karachi
Kuala Lumpur  Madrid  Melbourne  Mexico City  Nairobi
New Delhi  Shanghai  Taipei  Toronto

With offices in

Argentina  Austria  Brazil  Chile  Czech Republic  France  Greece
Guatemala  Hungary  Italy  Japan  Poland  Portugal  Singapore
South Korea  Switzerland  Thailand  Turkey  Ukraine  Vietnam

Oxford is a registered trade mark of Oxford University Press
in the UK and in certain other countries

Published in the United States
by Oxford University Press Inc., New York

British Library Cataloguing in Publication Data

Data available

Library of Congress Cataloguing in Publication Data
Betts, T. A. (Timothy Arnold)
  Epilepsy in women / Tim Betts, Harriet Clarke. — 1st ed.
    p. cm. — (The facts)
  Includes index.
  ISBN 978-0-19-954883-5
1. Epilepsy. 2. Women—Diseases. I. Clarke, Harriet. II. Title.
  RC372.B479 2009
  616.8'530082—dc22

                                                        2008036487

Typeset in Plantin
by Cepha Imaging Pvt. Ltd., Bangalore, India
Printed in China through
Asia Pacific Offset

ISBN 978-0-19-954883-5

10 9 8 7 6 5 4 3 2 1

# Foreword

As a woman who has grown from a teenager into a thirty something with epilepsy, the impact that it has had has, at times, dominated my life and the lives of those around me. However, for the most part, it has just been a background issue. Being diagnosed with epilepsy understandably raises lots of questions and frustratingly, there are not always answers to be had. The doctors that have treated me over the years have all been extremely knowledgeable with the information that they have available to them. Sadly, the specific issues that epilepsy raises in my life, both as an individual and as a woman, have not always been acknowledged or considered; this has occasionally made me feel as if the treatment I have been offered was a 'one size fits all' solution which can present problems.

I have asked questions regarding seizure control, personal safety, side effects, pregnancy, my ability to work, my driving licence and which anticonvulsant to try next to various healthcare professionals over the years. More often than not, it is a case of trial and error, prioritizing the issues and finding a balance. For example, does it matter if I put on a lot of weight if my seizures have stabilized? Does it matter that a drug may impact the development of a foetus in the future? Well of course it matters! However, the first priority of a neurologist treating epilepsy will always be to find a drug (or combination of drugs) that reduces or controls the seizures, therefore improving the health and decreasing the risk to the patient in front of them. This kind of scenario always leaves a slightly bitter taste—which I'm assured doesn't bypass the doctors—as you are grateful that you are one of the lucky ones and that your epilepsy has been controlled. However, the impact that the medication and the side effects can have on your life and health can almost be as damaging as the condition itself.

On a more positive note, it is refreshing to see that specific issues surrounding women and epilepsy are being given more attention and funding than there was just a few years ago. It is definitely something that I would have appreciated when I was newly diagnosed. As new research and literature becomes available, it is interesting to extend my knowledge which inevitably leads to a better dialogue with my doctors. Just when I think that I am a dab hand at epilepsy, a book like this one comes out and I learn something new. The statistics and research may not always provide good news but as with most situations in life, it is better to have an answer than none at all.

Sarah Lightbody, Eastcote, Middlesex

# Preface

Being a woman with epilepsy is not the same as being a man with epilepsy—menstruation, pregnancy, childbearing, and the menopause can affect epilepsy, and epilepsy and its treatment can affect menstruation, fertility, contraceptive choice and reliability, pregnancy and childbirth, parenting, and the menopause. So, a woman with epilepsy has much more to think about and more difficult treatment decisions to make than a man. Yet most books about epilepsy, whether for the professional or layperson, seem to be written with men in mind while the female perspective is either ignored or relegated to a separate chapter. Women, in addition to having some types of epilepsy exclusive to them, are, often for the reasons outlined above, less likely to achieve complete seizure control than men with epilepsy, even though men are slightly more likely to have epilepsy in the first place, but that's due to the fact that men are much more likely to sustain head injuries.

So, women with epilepsy deserve a book that adopts the female perspective from the start, and which describes in detail the problems that epilepsy can cause for them. Such a book should be equally helpful to, and understood by, both the woman with epilepsy and the professionals that work with her. It would be helpful if they and the patients they advise had the same understanding of the condition even if their perspectives are slightly different. But no book, no matter how detailed, can cover the whole range of epileptic experiences; all individual seizures and treatments must be discussed with a professional advisor; hopefully this book will be a guide to how this can be done.

We owe a particular debt of gratitude to those patients whose experiences, although deliberately jumbled to avoid identification (see brief vignettes scattered throughout the chapters), form one of the bastions of this book. We are also very grateful to three people—firstly, Kelly Jones who, as a layperson, has carefully read various drafts of this book and made some valuable suggestions which have hopefully added to its usefulness to the person with epilepsy who has suddenly had the illness thrust upon her; secondly, Witney Lau, a medical student, who has read various drafts as a professional reader to make sure it makes sense to that audience as well; and lastly Ben Cole who has kept Tim's computer knowledge in working order. If you read a vignette and think, 'hey, that's me', do remember that there is more than one person with epilepsy in the world and the vignettes have been chosen to illustrate universal truths about epilepsy and you, too, are part of that truth.

Tim Betts
Harriet Clarke

# Contents

# Part 1

# 1

# What is epilepsy?

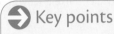

## Key points

- Epilepsy is a disorder of the brain and is comparatively common.
- It can occur in anyone, at any age: no one is immune.
- It is conventionally divided into those seizures that:
  - Start in the midbrain—primary generalized.
  - Start in the grey matter (the cerebral cortex)—partial seizures.
  - Start in the cortex and spread to the midbrain—secondarily generalized.
- Partial seizures are simple if consciousness is retained, complex if not.

## Three terms you need to know

- *ECG*—electrocardiogram. A device which, by means of electrodes stuck on the chest wall, records the electrical activity of the heart.
- *EEG*—electroencephalogram. A machine that records, via electrodes glued to the head, the electrical activity of the brain.
- *MRI*—magnetic resonance imaging. A modern method of imaging the structure of the brain; unlike computerized tomography (CT) imaging it does not use x-rays. An MRI angiogram looks at the blood vessels in the brain.

## How many people suffer from epilepsy?

Between 1 in 100 and 1 in 200 people will develop epilepsy at some time in their life (and 4–5% will have a seizure, often, but not exclusively, at the extremes of age without becoming 'epileptic'). That is a lot; indeed, epilepsy is the commonest serious brain disease to afflict mankind.

# The brain

Epilepsy starts in the brain. It is hard to conceive that this wrinkled, soft, pinky-grey lump is one of the most complex structures in the known universe. It contains billions of cells, endless connections both within and without the skull, all of our memories, present experiences, plans for the future, and our unique personalities.

Although we have to cut them apart to examine the brain, it and the spinal cord are really one organ. The brain is an organic whole and damage to part of it can have far-reaching consequences for the whole of it. A blow to one part of the skull likewise may cause injury in the opposite part of the brain—the so-called contre-coup effect—because in some ways the brain behaves like a jelly in a steel box when the head is struck.

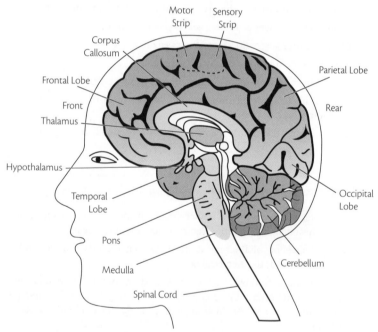

**Fig. 1.1** Brain cut through the middle from front to back

The brain consists of four separate but interconnected and interacting parts:

◆ The midbrain.

◆ The two cerebral hemispheres.

- The cerebellum.
- The spinal cord.

## Midbrain

The midbrain consists of bundles of 'white matter' (connective tissues running from the cerebral hemispheres to the spinal cord and vice versa, relaying information and commands) interspersed with embedded islands of grey (or brain) cells (the nuclei). The chief of these is the thalamus, the relay station between the cortex and the spinal cord; it is the seat of consciousness and an important site of epileptic activity. Lying just outside the brainstem is the hypothalamus, which, with the pituitary gland, regulates the cyclical supply of the hormones that control the phases of the menstrual cycle, amongst other functions.

## Cerebral hemispheres

The two cerebral hemispheres consist of a thin but much folded outer mantle, the cortex, with cells (neurons) lying in orderly rows, six cells deep and the inner white matter consisting of myriad bundles of connective tissue running to and from the other parts of the brain (including the other cerebral hemisphere via the corpus callosum) and the spinal cord.

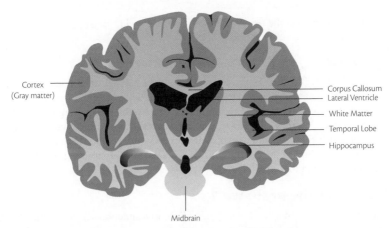

**Fig. 1.2** Cross-section from side to side through the middle of the brain

**Table 1.1** The parts of the cortex and their different functions

| Function | Area of the brain |
| --- | --- |
| Planning movements | Frontal lobes |
| Executing movements | Sensorimotor cortex (on opposite side) |
| Co-ordinating eye movement | Frontal lobes |
| Maintaining integrity of the personality | Mostly frontal lobes |
| Receiving bodily sensation | Sensorimotor cortex (on opposite side) |
| Reception of vision | Occipital lobes |
| Interpretation of what is seen | Temporal lobes |
| Receiving and analysing sound | Temporal lobes |
| Writing | Temporal and parietal lobes |
| Reading | Occipital and temporal lobes |
| Understanding and producing speech | Left temporal (mainly) and frontal lobe (even in most left-handed people) |
| Comparison of past and present experience | Temporal lobes (one of the elements of conscious awareness) |
| Formulation and storage of memory | Temporal lobes mainly |

Epileptic activity in the temporal lobes produces a wide variety of symptoms.

## Cerebellum

The cerebellum (the little brain) looks a little like a pickled walnut, and, as with the cerebral cortex, is divided into left and right lobes concerned with opposite sides of the body. Its main function appears to be the fine-tuning of muscle movements so that they are precise, smooth, and exact; one anticonvulsant drug (phenytoin) if taken to excess can cause irreversible cerebellar damage with resultant trembling of the hands, clumsiness, and difficulty walking (see Dora's case study later in this chapter).

# How does the brain work?

The answer is extremely complex (and still poorly-understood). All we need to briefly discuss here is how epileptic activity differs from ordinary brain activity. Let's start with a single brain cell (neuron). This is connected to other brain cells via processes called axons; these come from other neurons and terminate on our cell by means of connective plates called dendrites. The cell itself has its own connecting tube (or axon) with which it communicates with another cell. Dendrites 'speak' to the cells they are connected to by releasing very small amounts of special chemicals called 'neurotransmitters'. If sufficient is released, or the cell is primed, or other dendrites from other neurons are activated then sufficient energy is transmitted to our neuron and it 'fires'. In other words an electrochemical process travels down the axon to the next cell and a small amount of neurotransmitter is released which may (or may not) cause the next neuron to 'fire' in turn. There are different neurotransmitters some of which 'fire' the neuron, whilst others will switch it off; some are important in epilepsy and its treatment. After the neurotransmitter has been released, whether or not it activates the neuron, it is rapidly destroyed or reabsorbed back into the dendrite. This is happening all over the brain an incalculable number of times a second, even when we are asleep, mostly without our conscious awareness. It is a tightly organized process.

## So how is epilepsy different?

In an epileptic focus in the brain there is an, often small, group of cells (called the 'type 1 cells') that don't obey the usual 'firing' rules. They 'fire' repeatedly without regard to what is happening in the rest of the brain. This may pass unnoticed but occasionally spreads to the surrounding normal brain cells (the type 2 cells), which from time to time become caught up in this repetitive firing so that it spreads to involve enough of the brain to become noticeable as a seizure. What happens in the seizure depends on whereabouts in the brain this activity occurs and how far it spreads. Usually, since the brain contains its own, even if still little understood, restorative mechanisms it switches off again quite quickly, although the area of the brain where the firing occurred may not function properly for a while until it has fully recovered. Let's give a concrete example to explain.

### A sporting chance

You are playing football and you find yourself in front of the empty goal of the opposition with the ball at your feet and the goalkeeper out of position; you steady yourself, take aim, and with your right foot kick the ball into the back of the net. You may have thought about what you were doing but more likely you acted instinctively with conscious thought only switching on as you crash to the floor in a flurry of your ecstatic mates. Activity has gone on in millions of brain cells involving vision, hearing, balance, touch, and muscular activity involving complex tensing and relaxing.

## Harriet's seizure

My right leg rises up in exactly the same way it would to kick the football, except that I am alone in bed in the early morning: it gives a frantic kick, relaxes, kicks again, relaxes, and kicks again. I am wide-awake, frightened, but totally unable to control it. My right arm joins in with a couple of jerks of its own. I am still wide-awake, the jerking stops. I am left with a 'fuzzy' feeling in my right side and arm and leg are temporarily weak, although that soon wears off. Don't fuss!

That is a simple partial seizure (see Chapter 19).

There must be some kind of abnormality in the part of Harriet's brain where it all starts; but it is occurring in a valuable and vulnerable part of the brain so surgery, to remove the affected bit, might well cause too great a risk of irreparable damage. We must therefore control the abnormal cellular activity with medication, but the target we are trying to hit is very small and the risk of causing unpleasant side effects in the rest of the unaffected brain is high, as Harriet knows only too well (see Chapter 19).

## Three important points

- ◆ Type 2 cells are more likely to join in and 'fire' if the brain is fatigued, during the stages of sleep, episodes of stress or anxiety, or overbreathing.

- ◆ Once a seizure has occurred it 'sets up' the potential for the next one. For instance, structural and chemical changes take place in the brain and quiescent enzyme and genetic systems become active; this effect may last for a year and is one of the arguments for treating a first seizure (see Chapter 6).

- ◆ Certain female hormones are either proconvulsant (oestrogen) or anticonvulsant (progesterone); that is they make seizures more likely or less likely—see Chapter 9.

## Classification of seizures

Human beings have many different types of epileptic seizure. We are going to use the classification that your specialist will know and almost certainly use; suggestions are currently being put forward to modify or adapt it in the light of developing knowledge but have not yet been widely adopted.

Table 1.2 lists the primary generalized (or midbrain) seizures. We will discuss two in slightly greater detail.

### Simple (or typical) absence seizures

Simple (or typical) absences (previously called *petit mal*—the little illness) start and remain in the thalamus and are brief; since the thalamus is the seat of consciousness all that happens is that there is a short abrogation of conscious awareness which may sometimes be accompanied by rapid blinking or rhythmic jerking of the head and arms. The person does not fall and after a few seconds regains consciousness with no awareness that an attack has taken place. 'It's like being deaf in spots' as one patient explained. Although benign they need to be treated since even temporary lapses in consciousness can be dangerous. If they are not treated (or only inadequately) about a third to a half of the victims will at some stage develop tonic clonic seizures (see below), which are much more dangerous. They have a very characteristic EEG pattern (see Chapter 3) and can be readily induced by overbreathing (taking frequent deep breaths, more than are needed for quiet activity) so are easy to diagnose providing one has thought of the possibility.

**Table 1.2** Types of primary generalized seizure

| Type of seizure | Description | Age at onset | Pathology in brain | Treatment |
|---|---|---|---|---|
| Typical absence | Brief loss of consciousness; No awareness or memory | 10–14 years | Not usually | Usually successful |
| Atypical absence | Loss of consciousness with some awareness | Usually about 40 years | Not usually | Usually successful |
| Myoclonic | Repetitive jerks (arms, legs or both) Sometimes loss of consciousness | Usually teens | Sometimes genetic or brain damage | Depends on cause |
| Atonic | Sudden loss of muscle tone Loss of consciousness and falling | Usually teens | Not usually | Usually successful |
| Tonic | Sudden stiffening Loss of consciousness and falling | Usually teens | Not usually | Usually successful |
| Tonic clonic | Stiffening Loss of consciousness and falling Repetitive jerking | Any age | Sometimes genetic or brain damage | Depends |

## Tonic clonic seizures

Tonic clonic seizures (previously called *grand mal*—the big illness) are the epitome of epilepsy; what everybody thinks epilepsy is and is frightened by and the attack which those people who wish others to think that they have epilepsy attempt to imitate (usually not very successfully—see Chapter 4).

Tonic clonic seizures arise in the midbrain but can be triggered off by epileptic activity originating in the cortex. This gives rise to the frequently used description of the 'aura' followed by a tonic clonic seizure, a very common type of attack. 'Aura' is taken to mean warning but actually means breeze in ancient Greek.

There is a sudden loss of consciousness with stiffening of all the muscles of the body and falling with the ever-present risk of injury. This tonic phase is often accompanied by a characteristic cry as air is forced out of the lungs. The stiffening of the body is followed after a variable period by muscular relaxation followed by repetitive jerking, usually of the whole body—the clonic phase. This repetitive jerking eventually stops and there is often then another characteristic noise as air is drawn back into the lungs. This can be frightening to hear but is actually reassuring as it indicates that things are returning to normal—during the seizure itself breathing does not occur which is why people often go blue in the face (cyanosed) during an attack. Breathing may be noisy (and sometimes laboured) for a while as a lot of saliva and mucus can be produced during the attack; consciousness returns after a varying length of time. The person may be confused for some time afterwards until, often a little subdued, returning to her normal self.

### What can you do to help?

You can't stop the seizure but you can stay with the person protecting her from harm and concentrating on preventing damage to her head (using your cupped hands if necessary). When the seizure is over get her into the recovery position, lift the chin, and ensure that she can breathe (is the chest moving, is she 'pinking up'?) and stay with her until she has recovered her wits and knows where she is and how to get home or to where she wanted to go. Some women will have urinated during the attack and may want to find a lavatory to change in.

### Calling an ambulance

This is only rarely necessary but do so if:

- The seizure continues for more than 5 minutes.
- If she does not come round quickly when it is over.
- If she has obvious breathing difficulties or fails to start breathing again.
- You feel 'out of your depth' or your resuscitation skills are rusty.
- Remember, if it turns out to have been a false alarm the ambulance crew won't mind.

## Partial seizures

The symptoms experienced during a partial seizure are many and varied depending on whereabouts in the cortex it starts and how far it spreads. Not all of the experience will necessarily reach conscious awareness or be remembered after the attack (particularly if it ends in a tonic clonic seizure which can happen in about 50% of people with partial seizures). Partial seizures are usually fairly brief but it may take a longer time before brain function returns completely to normal (as in the case of Harriet). We call partial seizures in which consciousness is retained 'simple' and when it is not retained we call them 'complex'. Experiencing a simple partial seizure may be much more unpleasant for the person involved (ask Harriet).

## Frontal lobe epilepsy

### Seizure types

- May start with seizures that will not stop (so-called 'status epilepticus').
- Many secondarily generalize quickly so cortical origin not recognized.
- Frontal seizure discharge on one side may cause bilateral (both sides) movement.
- This movement may look wild and can be mistaken for mental illness.

- Apparent sexual behaviours may occur as part of the attack.
- Speech arrest, muttering, recognizable but out of context verbal phrases may occur.
- Frontal seizures are usually brief, may cluster, and often occur at night.
- There may be prolonged behaviour disturbance after the seizure is over.
- It can be tricky to tell (without EEG monitoring) if a seizure is frontal or temporal.

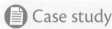 Case study

**Geraldine**, a 24-year-old, was near term with her first pregnancy when she began to be a little confused. This was thought to be due to a slightly raised blood pressure so she elected to have a Caesarean section. The confusion continued after the birth and she was clearly 'not herself'. She was given antidepressants and shortly afterwards, in the night, had a tonic clonic seizure in her sleep that did not stop. She was treated in her local hospital, returned home 2 days later having undergone no investigation and on a heavy dose of carbamazepine (an anticonvulsant).

She experienced no more tonic clonic seizures but was desperately tired; 3 or 4 times a week she would seemingly awaken, sit bolt upright and pound her thighs with her fists, swearing loudly for about 30 seconds. She would hit her husband if he tried to hold her: she would then tear off her nightdress and run downstairs crying uncontrollably, remaining confused and upset for half an hour before falling into a deep sleep.

She was seen in an emergency epilepsy clinic; video EEG monitoring revealed epileptic activity in both frontal lobes during a recorded seizure and an MRI scan showed a resolving haemorrhage in her right frontal lobe, presumably the remains of a small haemangioma (see Chapter 2) that had ruptured when her symptoms first started.

The antidepressant was stopped, levetiracetam (a different anticonvulsant) prescribed, and later the carbamazepine slowly removed; she remains seizure free and has recently had another baby.

## Sensorimotor epilepsy
### Seizure types

- Muscles of one hand alternately tensing and relaxing in a sinuous motion, slowly spreading up the arm to the shoulder (the 'Jacksonian march'); the leg may become involved or the attack die away. The patient is usually awake; a tonic clonic seizure may then supervene. The side on which it started may be weak for a short while afterwards (Todd's paralysis).

◆ A series of clonic jerks (see Harriet's seizure)—a tonic clonic seizure may follow.

◆ Tightening (tonic spasm) of limb(s), often prolonged and painful.

◆ Some seizures have sensory symptoms or there is a transient post-seizure change in sensory feeling (see Harriet's seizure).

◆ Focal (confined to one part of the body) tingling, numbness, or tickling (sometimes pleasant).

◆ Focal electric shock like sensations, pain, or burning feelings.

◆ Sexual sensations.

◆ Loss of feeling (anaesthesia).

◆ Body image disturbance (e.g. limbs seeming bigger).

◆ Some sensory seizures have a motor component, or there is post-seizure weakness.

◆ Some parietal lobe seizures are ignored until activity spreads elsewhere (see Cynthia's case study, below).

#  Case study

**Cynthia** was 18 and had just started at university when she began to get an odd, warm, and pleasant feeling in her left hand that also occasionally stiffened; it was only momentary, happening about twice a month and coincided with starting 'the pill' so she assumed it was just a side effect and did not discuss it with anyone. This went on for a couple of years until in her final year the feeling suddenly became more intense and frequent and was accompanied by stiffening and jerking of her whole arm. Initially this was put it down to 'exam stress' but Cynthia's parents noticed that she briefly lost consciousness during the episodes so she was seen urgently in an epilepsy clinic. She stopped 'the pill'.

Her left arm was weaker and less well co-ordinated than the right; an EEG (see Chapter 3) showed clear-cut spike wave activity in the right parietal-temporal area and an MRI angiogram (see Chapter 3) showed an arteriovenous malformation (see Chapter 2) of her right temporal lobe in which there had been a recent small bleed. This was successfully removed in a specialist surgical unit and she became seizure free, returning to university the following year to get a first-class degree. The weakness in her left hand and arm has gone. She currently takes levetiracetam (an anticonvulsant—see Appendix 1) and has restarted 'the pill'.

# Occipital lobe epilepsy
### Seizure types

- Unformed visual hallucinations (spots of colour, flashes of light).
- Transient loss of colour vision.
- Temporary loss of vision, usually in both eyes.
- Temporary double vision.
- Again, symptoms may be ignored until activity spreads further (see Amelia's case study, below).

##  Case study

**Amelia,** 61, a retired postal worker, was taking a diuretic (water relieving) drug for mild high blood pressure. She began to have 'odd spells' (her description) in which, although retaining consciousness, she would briefly feel 'odd and distant'. This feeling was accompanied by everything she looked at suddenly appearing in black and white; it went on for no more than a couple of minutes. She thought (as did her GP) that this was a side effect of her medication so it was changed.

However, the attacks became more frequent and intense and she began to be unable to speak during them (although she wanted to). She was referred and promptly investigated. Physical examination was normal apart from some loss of vision in the upper quadrants of her visual fields, suggesting a lesion in her left occipital lobe. MRI revealed a cystic lesion in this area; an initial EEG was normal, but a 24-hour EEG a week later captured a left occipital seizure spreading forward into the temporal lobe. When her history was taken again she remembered as a small child having a bad attack of measles which was followed for a couple of years afterwards by attacks of double vision, which disappeared of their own accord. The lesion was taken to be the result of previous measles encephalitis. The seizures completely resolved with a small dose of lamotrigine (an anticonvulsant—see Appendix 1) and she continues well.

# Temporal lobe epilepsy
### Seizure types

Temporal lobe seizures are the commonest type of epilepsy and there are many different types (see next page). They may be simple partial, complex partial, or initially partial followed by a tonic clonic seizure (which may wipe out the memory of what has happened before). The common types are listed in the box below.

## Seizures associated with phenomena related to the autonomic nervous system

- Intense sweating—generalized but sometimes localized.
- Intense whitening (or flushing) of the skin—usually the face.
- Sudden change in heart rhythm—slowing, speeding up, or irregular).

## Seizures associated with feelings out of keeping with the situation at the time

- Déjà vu—an intense feeling of 'I have been here before' when you haven't.
- Jamais vu—'I have never been here before' when clearly you have.
- Sudden intense fear.
- Sudden ecstasy.
- Sudden intense depression.
- Brief recurrent episodes of memory loss.
- Acute derealization—surroundings become meaningless and unreal.
- Depersonalization—intense feelings of personal unreality.
- Anger and aggression—sudden brief outbursts of extreme rage.

## Seizures associated with sensory phenonomena—almost always in one modality

- Visual hallucinations and illusions—often replay of a forgotten experience.
- Hallucinations of smell—usually, but not invariably, unpleasant or bizarre.
- Hallucinations of hearing—brief, intense, usually a single word or phrase.
- Hallucinations of taste—intense and often bizarre and unpleasant.
- Hallucinations of touch—by something unseen.

## Digestive experiences

- Intense nausea—rarely vomiting.
- A peculiar 'rising feeling' in the stomach area—very common

## Automatisms (stereotyped behaviour)—usually complex partial

- Lip smacking—very common.
- Chewing—often with, or following, lip smacking.
- Fumbling, scratching.
- Confused wandering.
- Undressing—rarely complete.
- Vocalization—usually single words or phrases, out of context.
- Motionless stare—often frightening in its intensity.

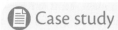 Case study

**Dora** was 22 and had had complex partial seizures since the age of 16. She would have a sudden loss of awareness plus incomprehensible muttering and attempted removal of her clothing for about a minute, but was confused and a little aggressive for about half an hour afterwards.

She was referred by her GP, who thought she might have a brain tumour, to a specialist unit. A previous EEG and CT scan had been reported as normal. She was taking a mixture of anticonvulsant drugs—phenytoin and valproate—but still had up to 3 seizures a week. She had become very unsteady on her feet and was unable to work or study because of severe tiredness.

A physical examination revealed signs of severe cerebellar damage. EEG monitoring and MRI scanning showed right temporal lobe seizures with right-sided hippocampal sclerosis (pre-existing damage) and marked loss of tissue in her cerebellum. She was taken off phenytoin because it can interact with valproate leading to permanent cerebellar damage (see Appendix 1), had successful temporal lobe surgery, and is now off all medication. She is taking an Open University degree and works as a nursing assistant. She still has some difficulty with balance and co-ordination but has learnt to compensate.

## Epilepsy found more commonly or exclusively in women

Some forms of epilepsy are more common in women, like childhood absence epilepsy and photosensitivity. Some seem to occur almost exclusively in women, like Rett syndrome, Aicardi's syndrome, and periventricular nodular heterotopia (see Chapter 2 for this latter form). This is possibly related to the presence of two X chromosomes in women (men have one X and one Y chromosome). About 12% of women only have seizures at a definite point in their menstrual cycle (see Part 2).

### Rett syndrome

The female child grows normally until about 1 year old and then rapidly regresses developmentally with the onset of frequent, usually intractable, atypical absences, partial and secondarily generalized tonic clonic seizures, stereotypical movements, and characteristic bursts of pathological laughter. The child survives (about 1 in 10,000 are affected) but ends up, as a young adult, severely mentally handicapped, usually unable to speak, walk, or use her hands. The mutated gene responsible for most cases of this condition (*MECP2*) also has a variant in mice and a recent study has shown that activating a normal copy instead of a mutated version of this gene in an affected mouse seems to reverse the symptoms; thus there is hope that something similar may be achievable eventually in humans.

## Aicardi syndrome

This is also known to be genetic in cause. From early on there are infantile spasms (seizures characterized by sudden generalized 'clenching' of the body) accompanied by either excessive muscular tone (spasticity), or (sometimes) loss of muscle tone (hypotonia), plus characteristic lesions (lacunae) to be seen in the back of the eye with an ophthalmoscope, and failure of the corpus callosum to develop (see Fig. 1.2) with associated severe learning difficulty.

## Photo and pattern sensitivity

About 5% of people with epilepsy (almost all with generalized epilepsy) are photosensitive—in other words exposed to flashing light of the right frequency they respond with epileptic activity in their EEG over the back part of the brain; the longer the flashing goes on, the more likely they are to have a seizure. So all people with epilepsy need to be thoroughly tested at least once for photosensitivity according to agreed international criteria (across the whole range of frequencies) and if they do show a positive response, then, according to what flicker rates they are sensitive to, they will need specific advice.

Some anticonvulsant drugs (valproate, lamotrigine, and levetiracetam) are effective against photo (and pattern) sensitivity, whereas others, such as carbamazepine, are not, so correct drug choice is essential. It is also necessary to determine whether the flashing light has to be seen in both eyes to induce a response (usually the case) or whether one eye is enough. If two eyes are involved and the person has only photically induced seizures, non-drug treatment (like Polaroid® spectacles) may be an option.

> Anyone with the condition should only watch television at least 10 feet (3 metres) away from the screen, have a light behind it, and always use the hand control to turn it off and on.

Many people with photosensitivity are sensitive to a flash frequency of 25 cycles per second which is a sub-harmonic of the alternating current supply of 50 cycles per second in the UK. In the USA the current supplied is at 60 cycles per second and relatively few people respond to the sub-harmonic of 30 cycles per second; it is very specific.

Up to 30% of people who are photosensitive are also pattern sensitive (exposed, usually in both eyes, to static or, more commonly, moving patterns of the right spatial dimensions they respond with epileptic activity and seizures—see the following case studies). This wasn't described until the mid 1950s although photosensitivity was known about even before the EEG was invented. Pattern sensitivity came into prominence with the development of computer games when some young people began to have seizures, usually for the first time, in front of their computer screen. At first it was put down to photosensitivity or the exotic nature of the programme but then it was realised that most were due to the person's visual cortex responding to the pattern being presented on the computer screen. Once this was recognized modern games were adapted so as not to have such patterns. Interestingly a species of ape has pattern-induced seizures; their predator is a leopard with a patterned coat, which, if seen in time, causes the ape to have a brief absence and drop to safety—why some human beings should have photo or pattern induced epilepsy is unknown. If you are not photosensitive you are very unlikely to be pattern sensitive.

## Animal epilepsies

Epilepsy is common in some animal species because it provides survival value. Tim has seen a rat (with sound-induced epilepsy), in a cage with a 'normal' rat, have a seizure when a bell was rung just outside the cage. Both rats took off running (since four-legged animals run in a tonic clonic seizure and don't fall over as a human would) and it was only when both were still again that Tim could tell the difference. One rat was awake and watchful again in its corner of the cage, the other clearly confused and temporarily 'out of it' in another corner. The unaffected rat walked stiff-legged up to the post-ictal rat and urinated on its head saying in effect 'I no longer recognize you as a rat'. After a few minutes the rat with epilepsy seemed to have joined the rat world again, leaving Tim to reflect that human and rat responses to a seizure were not that different—but had the affected rat been running from a predator it might well have escaped particularly because its flight path would have been unpredictable. Epilepsy is also common in dogs and there is a British Canine Epilepsy Society.

##  Case study

**June** and **Julia** were non-identical twins who went to university to study to be teachers. Both had been subject, since adolescence, to what had been called 'little faints' mostly whilst watching television (though in June's case sometimes elsewhere). These had been ascribed by their GP to their 'excitable natures' and had never been investigated. Shortly after arriving at university, June was standing in bright sunlight at a road junction. A procession of schoolgirls passed from left to right in front of her wearing bright hats that seemed to glow in the sunlight. Whilst watching them ('I seemed drawn to them' she explained) she had a tonic clonic seizure. Luckily there was a hospital nearby and after first aid she was given an appointment with a local epilepsy clinic.

She was seen with her sister; June had bursts of generalized epilepsy in her EEG on overbreathing and was both photosensitive (particularly at 25 cycles per second) and pattern sensitive. Julia had a normal EEG except that she was also photosensitive. June started on lamotrigine and became seizure free. Her EEG became normal with no photo or pattern sensitivity. Julia decided not to take medication but adopted the television precautions outlined, has a modern computer with a screen over the monitor and wears Polaroid® spectacles when driving. Both are now qualified teachers. For the rest of the family history see Chapter 2, Neuronal migration defects.

## Other 'reflex' epilepsies

These, like photo and pattern-induced seizures, are epilepsies induced by a specific, often very precise, stimulus (e.g. seeing an open safety pin causes a seizure whilst viewing a closed one does not). Reflex epilepsies are rare but important because they can sometimes be managed without recourse to anticonvulsants. Here are some examples:

### Simple reflex

- Flicker.
- Pattern.
- Tooth brushing.
- Touch—usually on a specific part of the body.
- Hot water immersion.

### Complex reflex

- Musicogenic—it is the tune and not the pitch or timbre of the music that induces the attack.
- Voice induced.
- Language or sound induced.

 Case study

**Maddie** was 15 and listening to a song on the radio whilst doing her homework when she overheard her father telling her mother that he was leaving home for good; she immediately had her first complex partial seizure and continued to have them despite much medication. It became clear to her eventually that seizures now only occurred when she heard the same song; unfortunately it was a popular song often heard on the radio or as incidental music in shops. She began to be afraid to listen to the radio or go out in case she heard it. She was referred for a second opinion.

It was decided to try to desensitize her to the tune; she was attached to an EEG machine and the tune played on a tape recorder continually. Epileptic activity appeared over her right temporal lobe and she then had a brief complex partial seizure: the tape continued. Another seizure occurred but took longer to arrive; when the tune continued to play further EEG activity occurred but no seizure came: the EEG abnormality then disappeared. Thereafter, providing she listened to the tune on a portable recorder for 5 minutes every day, no seizures occurred (she was taught a relaxation technique to accompany this). Her medication was reduced and discontinued after a further couple of years: she remains seizure free and no longer practises the listening exercise.

# 2

# The physical causes and emotional triggers of epilepsy

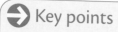

> ## Key points
>
> ◆ Over 60% of cases of epilepsy have no known cause.
> ◆ In some epilepsies, genetics is an important factor.
> ◆ It may be triggered by brain damage, blood vessel diseases, degenerative disorders, and alcoholism among other things.

A woman who suddenly develops, or eventually realises that she has, a potentially life changing and frightening condition like epilepsy will want to know why, and will turn to her doctor for support and information. Unfortunately, although epilepsy is common, we often do not know why a particular individual has acquired it. Indeed, a British study (in adult patients with newly diagnosed epilepsy) failed to find an identifiable cause for the epilepsy (after careful searching by acknowledged experts) in over 60%.

◆ Trauma (damage to the brain) 3%.
◆ Vascular (blood vessel related) 15%.
◆ Tumours (usually benign) 6%.
◆ Infections 2%.
◆ Degenerative (e.g. dementia) 6%.
◆ Alcohol 7%.
◆ Unknown cause* 61%.

(Figures taken from Sander, JW *et al.* (1990) *Lancet* **336**: 1267–71.)

The unknown percentage would be lower if we were only considering infantile epilepsy (where recognized and recognizable causes are much more common) or indeed epilepsy starting in old age (where cerebrovascular and other degenerative causes are more likely). There are two other points to be considered; firstly, epilepsy is comparatively common so sometimes another lesion will exist in the brain quite independent of the fact that the brain in question also has epilepsy. Secondly, some apparent causes of epilepsy, which in the past have almost been taken as read, may actually be comparatively uncommon or almost totally without foundation.

## ❌ Myths

❌ **Myth:** cerebral birth injuries cause much epilepsy.

❗ **Fact:** prospective studies suggest that this is an uncommon cause.

❌ **Myth:** febrile convulsions lead to later temporal lobe epilepsy.

❗ **Fact:** pre-existing temporal lobe abnormality leads to febrile convulsions.

❌ **Myth:** childhood immunization can cause epilepsy.

❗ **Fact:** apart from the occasional febrile convulsion, there is no evidence, in large-scale studies, that it does. It may even be protective.

# The known causes of epilepsy

## Genetic causes

There is little doubt that there is a genetic element to all epilepsy. In some well-defined syndromes like tuberous sclerosis (TS), it is of prime importance and we know the genes involved—mutations in either of two different genes seem to produce the same syndrome. In other syndromes like juvenile myoclonic epilepsy there is clearly a genetic element but several genes are involved in a complex way (multigenetic or polygenetic inheritance) and we are a long way from fully understanding it. But even in something like post-traumatic epilepsy there may be a genetic element; take one hundred soldiers with an identical head injury and only a proportion will develop epilepsy. Several contributing factors may be involved but one will be the individual's genetic predisposition toward epilepsy that has been awakened or switched on by the injury.

### Tuberous sclerosis

- This condition occurs in about 1 in 7000 live births and is dominantly inherited. This means that three out of four children of someone carrying the gene will inherit it but the syndrome may well not express itself fully so affected cases may not always be initially recognized for what they are (formes frustes).

- Many people with the disorder turn out to have a new gene mutation not previously present in the family and may be so mentally impaired that they are unlikely to pass the defective gene on.

- About 65% of those with one of the two genes known to independently give rise to TS will have epilepsy and around 40% will have significant learning difficulty.

- Seizures starting in infancy always lead to severe impairment of intelligence in TS.
- Behaviour problems and autism are common (but not invariable).

*The skin lesions*

- Red nodules on the face (angiofibromas)—may be hard to spot.
- 'Ash leaf' skin lesions, elsewhere, best seen under ultraviolet light.
- Fibrous skin plaques on forehead.
- 'Shagreen patches'—large areas of thick, discoloured skin—on the back (usually).

*Other lesions*

Characteristic lesions in the back of the eye (need ophthalmoscope to be seen).

'Candle guttering'—tubers on the walls of the lateral ventricles (see Figure 1.2). Seen on CT scans or MRI if radiologist knows TS suspected.

Benign, sometimes malignant, tumours in the brain.

- Usually benign tumours of the heart, kidneys, liver, bones, and rectum.

So, someone with the condition, or suspected of having it, needs careful assessment and it may be necessary to look at the parents and siblings and other close relatives. Excellent advice and information about TS can be obtained from TS Associations.

#  Case study

**Samantha** was 24 when she was first seen in a clinic. She was in a stupor (a rare side effect of her recently prescribed anticonvulsant tiagabine for her intractable epilepsy). She was taking four other anticonvulsants and was under the care of a local mental health service for severe learning difficulty (she did not speak) in addition to marked behavioural problems and obesity. She had never been investigated because of her aggressive behaviour. She was also taking two powerful antipsychotic drugs.

Physical examination revealed a weak and spastic right arm and leg and the characteristic lumpy red rash of TS on her face (which had not been remarked on before, being ascribed to her medication). She had a shagreen patch on her back and several ash leaf skin lesions. EEG initially suggested partial status (see Chapter 5) and MRI of her head showed two typical TS lesions adjacent to her left lateral ventricle. A year later, off all medication apart from two anti-convulsants, she was almost seizure-free, better behaved, had begun to speak and had lost 4 stone in weight. Physiotherapy had made her right side much stronger and she had a good relationship with her learning difficulty nurse. Examination of the rest of her family was normal, suggesting a new mutation.

## Juvenile myoclonic epilepsy

Juvenile myoclonic epilepsy is comparatively common (perhaps 10% of clinic referrals) and has a slightly muddled genetic element; indeed, in different studies in different countries, different gene sequences have been identified suggesting that it is not one uniform condition but perhaps several different ones that present in the same way. If one explores the extended family of an individual with the condition one usually discovers one or two relatives with similar epilepsy but also other family members who have generalized epileptic abnormalities in their EEGs but who do not have epilepsy; suggesting that something else has to happen to trigger the seizures off. Once they have started, of course, they tend to become self-perpetuating unless controlled by medication. Seizures usually start in early adolescence with myoclonic jerks, single or multiple, usually of the arms (sometimes one, sometimes both, and sometimes the legs) with or without brief (and often initially unnoticed) lapses of consciousness characteristically within the first hour after waking and often, in women, more severe premenstrually. They are equally common in men and women although women are more likely to be photosensitive. If untreated (as is often the case) at some time tonic clonic seizures will start to occur, again characteristically within the first hour of waking. Seizure frequency is made worse by sleep deprivation, too much alcohol, and stress (not the best news for the adolescent).

## A different sort of genetics—mitochondrial disorders

These disorders have come to prominence in the last 20 years, as scientists have begun to understand better how these essential components in the cell function. The mitochondria are small organelles contained within the neuron, the brain cell (along with the nucleus and cytoplasm). They possess their own genetic material—mitochondrial DNA—which is different from the DNA found in the cell nucleus and is inherited solely from the mother in both males and females, as mitochondrial DNA is derived entirely from the egg. The main function of mitochondria seems to be concerned with producing energy within the cell and much has been recently learnt about the rather complex disorders that can occur as a result of mitochondrial dysfunction (the mitochondrial encephalomyopathies—disorders of brain and muscle).

How a mitochondrial disorder presents clinically is complex and depends on the amount of abnormal mitochondrial DNA present and in which cells in the body it lies so a range of disability is possible; although specific syndromes have been described there is much overlap in symptoms (see below). The age at which a disorder first presents and can be recognized varies from childhood to early adult life. Two syndromes important in epilepsy are MERRF (myoclonic epilepsy with ragged red fibres—these fibres can be recognized under the microscope on muscle biopsy) and MELAS (mitochondrial encephalomyopathy, lactic acidosis with stroke-like episodes).

## MERRF

- Other maternally related relatives may have gene but be unaffected (or only partly).
- Myoclonus (muscular jerks) of all four limbs—often enough to prevent walking or feeding.
- Visual simple partial seizures with photosensitivity.
- Tonic clonic seizures.
- Deafness.
- Short stature.
- Loss of intellect.
- Multiple benign fatty tumours (lipomas).

## MELAS

- Other maternally related relatives may have gene mutation but be apparently unaffected.
- Early development often normal then epilepsy supervenes (partial or generalized with some myoclonus).
- Recurrent headaches and vomiting.
- Loss of intellect (not invariably).
- Muscle weakness.
- Deafness.
- Short stature.
- Lactic acidosis (excess amounts of lactic acid in the blood stream).
- Characteristic stroke-like episodes that start in early adult life.

## Developmental disorders

### Cysts (dermoid and epidermoid)

Cysts are derived from skin elements (there is a close relationship in the developing fetus between skin and nervous tissue), can be found in brain tissue, and are not malignant (that is they do not grow) but can, by their effects on surrounding cells, become the focus for epileptic activity. Often, but not invariably, they can be removed surgically partly to be sure of the diagnosis and partly because after a couple of years, if removing the cyst stops the epilepsy, then anticonvulsants can usually be safely slowly withdrawn which may be important in women planning pregnancy.

## Neuronal migration defects

Neuronal migration defects are a not uncommon cause of epilepsy although their full significance is still being established as MRI scanning becomes more usual. There are several types with rather jaw-breaking names but all derive from the somewhat complicated development of neurons (brain cells); indeed, if one studies neuronal development in detail one wonders how it ever goes right.

Basically neurons originate, whilst the human baby is still in the womb, in the middle of the developing brain and then 'migrate' along set pathways to lie (as the grey matter) in orderly rows, six cells deep, on the outside of the brain which becomes much convoluted (or folded) to accommodate them. They then develop complex interconnections and it is the number and richness of these connections that partly determines how intelligent the owner of the particular brain appears to be. About twice as many neurons migrate to the outside of the brain than are needed, so, after making the journey, half then die and disappear. If the neurons don't arrive at their destination or don't disappear when they should, the brain has a problem (bearing in mind that the infant brain is to some extent 'plastic' so that other areas of the brain can sometimes take on the function of missing neurons).

### Types of neuronal migration defect

- *Schizencephaly*—a deep cleft in the motor and sensory area lined by usually disorganized cells; if just on one side little may be apparent; learning difficulty if on both sides.

- *Hemimegalencephaly*—too many neurons jammed together (polymicrogyria) with severe epilepsy, paralysis, and loss of intellect.

- *Lissencephaly*—loss of migrated neurons with haphazard cortical organization (agyria, microgyria), severe learning difficulty, and epilepsy: known to be inherited.

- *Pachygyria*—the opposite of polymicrogyria; scattered areas in the brain where neurons have failed to migrate properly with resultant learning difficulty.

- *Nodular heterotopias*—isolated and disconnected islands of neurons in the white matter; may be familial (see Case study—June and Julia (again)).

- *Laminar heterotopia*—so-called 'double cortex' with separate inner and outer layers; found only in women, usually associated learning difficulty and epilepsy.

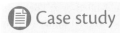 Case study

**June and Julia (again).** Perhaps because it had taken so long to realise that June and Julia had epilepsy plus some other health anxieties the immediate family requested if they could be assessed, which was accordingly done. On MRI scanning June had been shown to have an incidental nodular heterotopia (on the left side; she was left handed), Julia's scan was normal. Their mother had a normal scan but had traces of generalized epilepsy in her EEG, but was not photo or pattern sensitive (but, of course may have been in the past; she had never had a seizure that she knew of). Tom, the older brother, had a normal scan and EEG; Jennifer, the younger sister, had a normal scan but her EEG showed she was photo sensitive at 25 cycles per second (like her sisters) but not pattern sensitive. She decided to take the same TV-watching precautions as her sisters (but not the Polaroid spectacles—'ugh' she said). The father had a normal EEG but, like his daughter June, had a nodular heterotopia on the left side on MRI scanning (he was also left handed). Careful neurological examination of both June and her father revealed no abnormality. It looks as though June has possibly inherited a mutated gene from both sides of the family, but neither should give her any further trouble.

## Corpus callosum

The corpus callosum (see Figure 1.1) is sometimes missing in epilepsies associated with learning difficulty and occasionally lack of a corpus callosum exists as an isolated defect without other abnormalities in association with epilepsy. It is said in such cases that the epilepsy is due to loss of inhibitory activity; this may be so but why, if that is true, do surgeons actually cut the corpus callosum to treat otherwise intractable epilepsy with some success? Possibly because surgeons do not divide more than two-thirds of it; possibly for other reasons that we, as yet, do not understand.

## Intrauterine and perinatal injury (anoxia)

The association between anoxia (lack of oxygen) in the womb and in the first few months after birth and epilepsy is now known not to be very strong because controlled studies have shown that the incidence of cerebral birth injury in people with early onset epilepsy is little different from that in people who do not have epilepsy, and febrile convulsions are due either to a pre-existing propensity to epilepsy or the result of damage already in the brain. There is a relationship between cerebral palsy or learning difficulty and epilepsy but these are not often caused by cerebral birth injury. There is also a relationship between thrombosis (clotting) in one of the cerebral arteries, usually occurring during birth, and epilepsy (which sometimes does not develop until many years later), the site of the original injury being represented by a fluid-filled cyst. The child or adolescent may have no discernible symptoms of the original injury or may have one-sided motor and sensory weakness and loss.

## Infections

Encephalitis (infection and inflammation of the brain substance itself, usually viral) and meningitis (inflammation of the membranes that surround the brain which may be due to bacterial or viral infection) are potentially very serious and relatively common infections in childhood and early adult life. Both may be the cause of enduring epilepsy particularly if the person has seizures during the acute stage of the illness or, after recovery from it, continues to have symptoms or signs suggestive of brain damage. This subsequent epilepsy may be difficult to control particularly if, as is sometimes the case, it originates in more than one site in the brain. Other newer infections may cause seizures and need nowadays to be thought about; acquired immune deficiency syndrome (AIDS) may present initially with epilepsy as may the new form of Creutzfeldt–Jakob disease (myoclonic jerks), but without the very characteristic EEG changes that occur in the older form of this disorder (which still exists and can also cause epileptic seizures). In other parts of the world diseases such as tuberculous meningitis or cysticercosis (a parasitic disease of the brain) are common causes of post-infective epilepsy.

## Trauma

(Also see *Head Injury: The Facts*, another book in this series.) By and large, brain trauma only causes epilepsy if it is severe and leaves behind damage or scarring, such as after a depressed skull fracture or a penetrating injury to the brain; here the risk of subsequent epilepsy is high (though by no means inevitable) and persists for some years after the injury. The risk of seizures after a head injury is also increased if there is a long period of post-injury loss of memory (but this, of course, suggests brain injury) or if seizures occur in the first week after the injury (but that, again, suggests brain injury).

Do less severe cases of head injury (no depressed skull fracture, no obvious brain penetration or discernable scarring, or immediate seizures) lead to subsequent epilepsy? Careful large-scale follow up studies have suggested that the risk, in such circumstances, is very small. It is also possible that the head injury that supposedly caused the epilepsy was actually the first (but unrecognized) seizure itself. If minor head injury does sometimes lead to epilepsy it is likely (as with febrile seizures) that the patient was already predisposed to epilepsy and the head injury was the last straw in a complicated chain of inevitable events. If you already have epilepsy then even a mild head injury can precipitate a flurry of post-injury seizures that may persist for a few weeks.

## Blood vessel diseases

These are a not uncommon cause of epilepsy (although they may also occur in the brains of people who do not have epilepsy) and there are several kinds.

The blood supply to (and venous drainage from) the brain is quite complex and, in places and particularly in some vulnerable individuals, arterial walls are thin or even deficient so balloon out and rupture quite readily under increased pressure (such as the raised blood pressure that can go with increasing age) or after relatively minor injury. Blood supply to the brain comes from the carotid arteries in the front of the neck (that meet in a circle around the midbrain) and a posterior supply from the vertebral and basilar arteries at the back of the brain that eventually also meet the circle.

## Cavernous haemangiomas

These are small cysts (sometimes calcified), which probably originate from small malformed blood vessels in the brain substance. They may rupture (see the Case study of Geraldine in Chapter 1) and can usually be removed surgically if the epilepsy does not respond to medical treatment.

## Arteriovenous malformations

These can occur anywhere in the brain and may be small or sometimes very large. They are basically a deformity of the usual junction between arteries and veins in the brain and are particularly likely to rupture causing bleeding, which can be very damaging. They are often associated with epilepsy and, if found when the epilepsy is first diagnosed (they show up well on MRI scanning) their future management needs to be discussed with a neurosurgeon as it may be safer to remove them if possible (not necessarily to treat the epilepsy). Other surgical approaches to block them off can also be tried: it is important to make sure that the patient's blood pressure is well controlled.

## Aneurysms

Aneurysms occur in the blood supply to the brain where there is a congenital weakness in the arterial wall (usually failure of the elastic lining to develop properly) and are sometimes associated with focal epilepsy. As a result of blood pressure playing on the weakness the arterial wall balloons out and may eventually give way with a resulting drastic and damaging haemorrhage; sometimes before it gives way the swelling puts pressure on surrounding cranial nerves running close by so that neurological signs come and go (like, for instance, an enlarged pupil on one side or a recurrent squint). About 5% of the population are said to have potential cerebral aneurysms; most never give trouble; some rupture without warning and some rupture after giving warning signs that, for one reason or another, are ignored.

## Stroke

(Also see *Stroke: The Facts*, another book in this series.) Strokes are particularly common in the older population, but not confined to them. There are two basic kinds of stroke, cerebral haemorrhage (bleeding, when a blood vessel in the brain actually ruptures as do aneurysms as mentioned above) and cerebral thrombosis (when a blood clot blocks off a cerebral artery somewhere in the brain). A transient ischaemic attack (TIA) is a brief stroke-like episode that swiftly recovers—but is a warning that all is not well in the brain's blood supply.

Up to 10% of people who have a stroke will then or later develop epilepsy. Unlike with brain injury the severity of the stroke seems unimportant in deciding whether the person will develop epilepsy or not and many people who have TIAs also develop concomitant epilepsy indicating quite widespread blood supply impairment in the brain. It is usually possible in the older person to control stroke or impaired blood supply-related epilepsy with medication although it is better, if possible, to avoid anticonvulsant medication that has too many interactions with other drugs which the patient will probably also be taking. This control, however, takes time and patience on both the patient's and doctor's part which some older people don't receive.

## Tumours

❌ Myth

❌ **Myth:** if you develop epilepsy you've probably got a brain tumour.

❗ **Fact:** only 6% of people with newly diagnosed epilepsy have a tumour and it is usually benign.

Although benign (slow growing or static) tumours are an important if not very frequent cause of epilepsy (in a recent audit of people with epilepsy seen in the Birmingham University Seizure Clinic only 6% had tumours, almost all benign, exactly the same percentage as in the earlier London survey), malignant (rapidly growing, spreading) tumours are not; even if a malignant tumour does present with epilepsy almost invariably other signs and symptoms that indicate the true diagnosis will also be present (see the Case study of Julie in this chapter). However, some benign tumours, indolent for years, may suddenly start to grow or have a bleed into their substance, which may confuse and complicate diagnosis and management. So, in general terms and if to do so is safe, most patients and most doctors would want the tumour surgically removed and under the microscope (at least a piece of it) to be certain of its nature. Removing the tumour may also in the fullness of time mean that the patient can withdraw from their anticonvulsant medication.

Here are two other points about tumours:

◆ Malignant tumours elsewhere in the body (cancers) can spread (metastasize) to the brain, particularly lung cancer in men (and some women) and breast cancer in women (and the occasional man) and cause seizures. Although this is grim news to receive it is often possible nowadays to at least extend a useful and comfortable life in such patients.

◆ A particular type of tumour, its importance, and relative commonness as a cause of epilepsy unrecognized until the advent of MRI scanning (which picks it up with relative ease) is the (wait for it!) dysembroplastic neuroepithelial tumour. Its importance lies in the fact that it is a relatively common cause of intractable focal epilepsy and that (often unseen on a CT scan) on an MRI scan it often looks malignant, but actually isn't–and can often be removed safely.

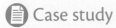 Case study

**Julie** had a normal birth, development, and schooling. She passed her driving test at the first attempt at 17 and left school a year later with three good 'A levels' to become a teaching assistant, a job which she loved, and married a soldier at 25 intending to have her first child at 30 when he left the army. An uneventful, happy life. At 27 she began to have brief episodes of confusion initially put down to worry about her husband serving abroad. The attacks swiftly progressed however, to be followed after a couple of months by brief tonic clonic seizures and she began to have intense left-sided early morning headaches so she was referred for an urgent appointment.

Physical examination revealed a weak and slightly spastic right arm and leg and a swollen optic disc (a sign of raised intracranial pressure); an EEG showed marked slowing and epileptic activity over the left temporal lobe and an MRI revealed a large aggressive looking left temporal lobe tumour. A neurosurgeon in a delicate operation 'debulked' as much of the growth as he could but had to leave some behind, as it was too dangerous to remove because of the risk of irreparable neurological damage. She had some radiotherapy and feels much better although still has some brief complex partial seizures. She knows the growth may return and has been taught to recognize the early signs of recurrence and has yearly MRIs. Despite the risk she has gone ahead with her first pregnancy and plans to have another; her husband got an early discharge from the army to be with her: 'every cloud has a silver lining' she says. She is one of the bravest people Tim has ever known.

## Learning difficulty

Some people with epilepsy also have learning difficulty (problems with acquiring the skills and knowledge needed to get through life unaided). Sometimes this is because the individual lacks specific skills (as in dyslexia), which do not impair her general level of intelligence but make it more difficult for her to express it, until ways round the problem are learnt. Sometimes learning difficulty occurs because the person's general level of intelligence is low. Intelligence in the human population lies on a normal distribution curve from very high to very low, with very few individuals at either end of the extremes and most of us bunched in the middle; but the bottom end is slightly skewed by those whose limited intelligence is caused or augmented by early acquired brain damage or genetic conditions (as, for instance, tuberous sclerosis—see the Case study of Samantha earlier in this chapter). Although there is no direct relationship between intelligence and epilepsy in that epilepsy is equally likely to occur in those of high intelligence as in those of low, it is more likely to occur in those with lack of intelligence caused by some specific condition (as with Samantha) as the condition that causes the impaired intelligence also causes the epilepsy.

## Dementia

Dementia is a brain illness in which there is a progressive loss of intellectual power, sometimes slow, sometimes rapid, sometimes episodic depending on the cause of the illness and to be distinguished from the slow decline in some aspects of intellectual powers normal in old age. About 10% of people with Alzheimer's disease (the commonest form of dementia in the UK) and cerebrovascular dementia (the second commonest) will develop (often partial) seizures as part of their illness. These are often comparatively easy to treat but may unfortunately pass unrecognized or are ascribed to other causes. In this regard it is important to recognize that, if the epilepsy comes first, the progressive subsequent intellectual decline in the patient is nothing to do with the epilepsy itself. It is important to exclude other treatable conditions and not just ascribe any intellectual loss in old age to Alzheimer's dementia. Other rare forms of dementia (such as Pick's disease) may also have epilepsy as part of their clinical picture as can the dementia sometimes associated with AIDS.

### So-called 'pseudodementia'

This is a condition that looks superficially like a dementing illness and the patient 'written off' in consequence when the real culprit is an unrecognized removable tumour or remediable but unnoticed drug intoxication. Depression in the elderly can also look uncommonly like dementia; to this day Tim remembers an elderly lady on one of the psychogeriatric wards of a Midland mental hospital whose demented mutterings he was idly listening to as he had a cup of tea with the nurses until he realised that the mutterings were those of guilt, self accusation, and unworthiness; 3 weeks later, with some antidepressants inside her, a no longer hopelessly confused but now sprightly old lady was at the door demanding to go home, much, it is sad to relate, to the dismay of her relatives who were already planning the disposal of her property.

## Metabolic conditions

In infants and very young children metabolic disorders (like genetic disorders) may be an important cause of epileptic seizures outside the compass of this book but worth discussing with a paediatric neurologist.

In adults other metabolic conditions are a rare but important cause of seizures:

◆ *Hypoglycaemia*—low blood sugar, due to disease of the pancreas.

◆ *Raised blood urea*—failing kidneys, seizures sometimes the first symptom.

◆ *Raised calcium*—disorder of the parathyroid glands in the neck.

This demonstrates the importance of carrying out a 'biochemical profile'—about twenty biochemical blood tests—on every person with new-onset epilepsy to pick up these rare causes and also to detect the effect that anticonvulsant drugs can sometimes have on blood chemistry.

## Alcohol

◆ *Rum fits*—too much alcohol leading to intoxication and a flurry of seizures.

◆ *Sudden withdrawl*—leads, in the habituated to delirium tremens and, in 50%, to a burst of epileptic seizures. This can be fatal and needs urgent treatment.

◆ *Chronic alcoholism*—leads in some to chronic, difficult to treat, epilepsy, unless the patient can be encouraged to become, and stay, 'dry'.

The good news is that if you have epilepsy you usually don't have to stop drinking (very rarely even a very small amount of alcohol does seem to induce a seizure; if that is the case for you then you will have to get used to a life without it). For most of you, providing you don't overindulge at any one time and stick to the safe and sensible limits (no more than 15 units of alcohol a week) remembering that a small—and we do mean small—glass of wine is 1 unit. Half a pint of beer is also 1 unit. Its also a good idea to have two or three alcohol-free days a week so that your body and your brain gets used to being without alcohol from time to time; but also don't down all your weekly allowance in one fell swoop at the weekend; your friends won't like it and neither will your epilepsy (or you, or your purse, the next morning).

## Other poisons

We hope it goes without saying that you should studiously avoid the other substances that most young people seem to be offered as soon as they set foot outside their front door. It is just not safe if you have epilepsy; so just say (and keep saying, with conviction) no.

Your doctors, too, may offer you medication for conditions other than epilepsy; it is worth checking with them that what is being offered is safe as far as your epilepsy is concerned and will not interfere with (or be interfered by) the medication you are taking for your epilepsy. Some psychotropic drugs (used for emotional complaints), particularly some antidepressant drugs, can indeed trigger off seizures in people who don't have epilepsy and worsen the frequency of seizures in those who do have it—see the Case study of Geraldine in Chapter 1—and the efficacy of other drugs, like antibiotics, may be slightly reduced (so you need a bigger dose) if you are taking an anticonvulsant drug which is markedly enzyme-inducing (see Chapter 7 and Appendix 1 for further information). And don't forget to ask about the pill and your anticonvulsant medication—let's hope your doctor knows the answer or has the sense to check. And, as we say in Chapter 6, don't take benzodiazepine tranquillizers if you have epilepsy except for epilepsy itself; if you have anxiety problems then behavioural or cognitive counselling would be much safer and probably, in the long run, more efficacious.

## States of mind, stress, and epilepsy

There is no doubt that the way you feel, particularly how anxious you are, can affect the frequency of your seizures (in a few people we have known it seems to be the other way round; highly aroused they are seizure free, it is when they relax that the seizures start). Most people when they are anxious (and there is nothing quite like epilepsy to make you anxious) breath more quickly than they need to—the technical term is overbreath—which increases the likelihood of a seizure. States of mind can also directly induce a seizure although this is not common, but over breathing related to anxiety about seizures is, and commonly precipitates seizures in those people with epilepsy who are stressed so that stress management has a place in the management of some people with epilepsy.

## Women's matters

Likewise being a woman, subject to regularly fluctuating tides of hormones both during her periods and later during the early days of the perimenopause and menopause, can have its own effects on seizures and seizure frequency (at least 12% of women seem to have most of their seizures during the week before their periods, for instance) and deserves a section of the book to itself, so see you in Part 2.

# 3

# How epilepsy is diagnosed—or should be

## → Key points

- The diagnosis of epilepsy is based on the account of the attack(s) given by the victim and any witnesses to a doctor or specialist nurse.
- This can easily lead to mistakes in diagnosis for various reasons.
- Nowadays it is sometimes possible to record attacks on continuous EEG and video monitoring; this aids diagnosis.
- Once the diagnosis is made various investigations are done to try to determine the cause (like ECG, EEG, and MRI).

It is not always easy to diagnose epilepsy: there is no doubt that some people given the diagnosis and started on treatment do not actually have it and that some people, given a different diagnosis, eventually turn out to have epilepsy or a different type than that originally diagnosed. There are several reasons for this.

- The person who makes the diagnosis very rarely sees the seizure.
- She or he has to rely on the account of the patient (who may recall nothing) and the account of a witness who may have been terrified and may not describe or remember important points but wants to get across how frightened he or she was—something that unless talked through may leave a dissatisfied patient and family.
- Other distortions may occur if the witness has some medical knowledge, like the dentist who reports a faint as 'an obvious tonic clonic seizure' or doctors and nurses, unused to the wide varieties of epileptic experience, who will tend to report what they think they ought to have seen, rather than what they actually did.
- So in considering the diagnosis of epilepsy we should think in terms of a hierarchy of investigation.

# The medical history

'Listen to the patient; she is telling you the diagnosis' is an old (but still true) medical adage. As full an account as possible of the seizures (and what happens before and after them) must be obtained from the person who has them and any witness (whose account is invaluable particularly in the case of a child or a person with communication difficulty to flesh out the history—but it is also very important not to exclude the child (or impaired adult) from the conversation). There follows:

## A general medical and psychiatric history

- History of pregnancy and birth.
- Any genetic traits in family (including seizures)?
- Any past illnesses?
- Checklist of symptoms relevant to each body part (brain, heart, abdomen, urinary, etc.).
- Any history of brain injury or infection?
- Any undue depressive or anxiety symptoms? Any psychotic symptoms?
- What medication is being taken (including 'the pill' or contraceptive injections).
- How much alcohol do you drink? (Doctors usually record double the amount you say).
- Do you use illicit drugs (asked tactfully)?

## An example—headache

Enquiry will be made about any headaches or episodes of vomiting that the patient may have had. Headaches are a common symptom (tension, migraine, and sinus infection being the commonest causes) and each tend to have their own characteristics although distinguishing between them is not always easy (of course, since they are common, the patient may have more than one type; many people with migraine, not unsurprisingly, have tension headaches and, to avoid overtreatment of the migraine—which, in itself can lead to headache—it is important to recognize the difference between them).

## Symptoms of different types of headache

- *Migraine* Episodic; may be characteristic warning symptoms—one-sided; nausea and/or vomiting; blurring or loss of vision during attack (often one-sided); may be accompanied by transient one-sided weakness or loss of sensation; responds well to appropriate anti-migraine medication.

◆ *Sinusitis* Usually continuous during episodes; around forehead and front of face; may be raised temperature, sometimes nausea; sometimes purulent nasal discharge.

◆ *Tension* Varies in intensity; usually worse on forehead, temples, or back of head; situational; may be nausea; may be accompanying depression so may be apparent changes in memory or mental powers (particularly if patient frightened by symptoms).

◆ *Cerebral tumour* (Remember this is rare; see Case study of Julie, Chapter 2.) Sometimes one-sided; characteristically worse in early morning; may be nausea and vomiting; blurring of vision common; may be continuous one-sided weakness or loss of sensation; slow growing tumours may have no symptoms at all as brain 'accommodates' them; may be changes in memory or mental powers.

# The medical examination

It is usual to then perform a physical examination, which may be extensive or not (depending on what has been said in the medical history). It is usual to record a blood pressure and sometimes to look at the back of both eyes with an ophthalmoscope seeking the signs of raised intracranial pressure (swelling in part or all of the brain—see the Case study of Julie, Chapter 2).

## Blood tests

It is usual on the first visit to carry out some screening blood tests including those for anaemia plus various biochemical tests that can suggest specific bodily disorders such as raised blood calcium (see Chapter 2). Other blood tests may be indicated by the patient's history and examination (e.g. glandular fever).

## Special tests

At this stage, having taken a careful history and performed whatever physical examination is felt to be necessary, it is usually possible to make a diagnosis or, if that is not possible, to decide what other steps will be necessary. The special tests that follow are not primarily for diagnosis, with the exception, sometimes, of ECG and EEG monitoring and a plasma prolactin level.

### The electrocardiograph (ECG)

Anyone with suspected epilepsy should have a 12-channel ECG; some people have seizures which are assumed to be epileptic but which are actually cardiac in origin (see the Case study of Fiona in Chapter 4) and which, untreated, can be fatal. With prolonged ECG recording it is now possible to 'catch' a seizure; indeed one device can record continually for several weeks at a time (preserving the record if an attack occurs) and, although somewhat expensive, can be invaluable in making a diagnosis. Sadly, until recently, those doctors that deal with disorders of the heart (cardiologists) and those that deal with disorders of the brain (neurologists and neuropsychiatrists), both of whom are faced with the problem of patients that suddenly lose consciousness, have communicated but little with each other.

## The electroencephalogram (EEG)

The first special investigation for epilepsy is the EEG. Since an ordinary EEG only monitors about 20 minutes of brain activity on a particular day it may well be of little value, as a normal EEG does not mean that the patient does not have epilepsy and an abnormal EEG does not necessarily mean that she does. An EEG trace is recorded from electrodes glued on the head.

- *Alpha* rhythm—basic rhythm with the eyes shut (over the back part of the head).
- *Theta* rhythm—(slower) appears if the patient is drowsy.
- *Delta* rhythm—(very slow) appears when the patient is asleep. When the patient is dreaming there is also a characteristic EEG pattern.
- *Spike and wave*—the rhythm seen in epileptic discharge.

If an adult patient is clearly awake then theta and delta activity is abnormal (particularly if in only one part of the EEG). Spike and wave can be generalized (typical absences have a very diagnostic generalized 3 per second spike wave pattern) or partial (occurring in only one part of the EEG). A basic EEG usually has a period of vigorous over breathing (which can bring out epileptic activity) and photic (flashing light) and visual pattern testing (see case study of June, Chapter 1). An EEG recorded immediately after a seizure can be helpful if it shows a typical post seizure pattern.

## The sleep EEG

If the basic EEG is normal it is usual to then carry out a sleep EEG, as abnormalities may appear that are not seen in an ordinary EEG. Some EEG departments merely record an EEG for about half an hour with the patient not having slept the night before (not the easiest thing to achieve if you are not used to it, although all-night television has made it easier) and staying awake during the recording (a sleep-deprived EEG which may yield valuable information). Other departments ask the patient not to sleep as already described, record a sleep deprived EEG, but then let the patient fall asleep for a few hours so that the EEG has recorded sleep deprivation, falling asleep, the stages of sleep and waking up again; this latter approach is more likely to record abnormality (and is particularly important if the patient only has sleep related seizures) but requires the EEG department to have a quiet room in which EEG and video recording can take place away from the bustle and conversations of a busy department.

## Prolonged EEG recording

Sometimes it is important to record a seizure on EEG (either for diagnosis or to accurately localize seizures for possible surgery) and two methods are used to try to achieve this. Indeed, as better methods are now available for visualizing the brain and its function (see later in this chapter) this is becoming an ever increasing and more important diagnostic role for the EEG department as far as epilepsy is concerned.

The first method is ambulatory EEG recording. Electrodes are securely glued to the head and attached to a portable EEG recording device (worn in a small bag, usually over the shoulder) and the patient then goes home. The device can record for up to 24 hours at a time. The great advantage of this method is that seizures are more likely to occur in the patient's home environment. The disadvantages are that a video record of the attack may not be obtained and the number of electrodes is limited so that accurate localisation of the attack may be difficult. Some authorities decry this method and don't use it, but it is comparatively cheap. A basic ECG rhythm strip can also be recorded or a more elaborate ECG recording device can be added separately.

The other method is to bring the patient into the EEG laboratory and record video and (with a full number of electrodes) EEG and ECG signals continually for several days and nights. Sometimes medication is partly or wholly withdrawn. The main problems with video-EEG monitoring are ensuring that seizures are actually recorded which often means booking patients in at a time when seizures are most likely to occur (e.g. premenstrually), trying to ensure that the patient's seizures don't just occur when they are out of sight whilst on the lavatory or washing, and being able to justify the not inconsiderable cost. Such monitoring is, however, essential if surgery is contemplated and is also extremely useful to make an accurate diagnosis of the nature of a patient's seizures (which may not, of course, be epileptic—see Case study of Emily, Chapter 4).

## Magnetic resonance imaging (MRI), computed tomography (CT), and positron emision tomography (PET)

Since there are several possible structural or physical causes of epilepsy (which may not be revealed by the history, physical examination, or EEG) it is important to carry out imaging of the brain and its substance. This is best done by a high quality MRI scan of the brain, configured for epilepsy (i.e. to show the temporal lobes and hippocampi clearly). Sometimes magnetic resonance angiography (looking at the blood vessels) is also needed. If MRI is not readily available some authorities suggest CT scanning (computer-controlled multiple x-rays of the head which give an enhanced image compared with a single x-ray—but, of course, more radiation), but this can fail to reveal much that is clearly revealed by MRI scanning including hippocampal sclerosis. Some people find being in an MRI scanner claustrophobic and unpleasant and for them prior sedation with a drug like diazepam may be advisable (though some MRI scanners are more open and less terrifying). Most scanners, too, have a weight limit for patients so the very overweight patient often has to travel a couple of hundred miles to find a scanner that can accommodate her.

MRI scanning does not expose the patient to potentially harmful radiation whereas CT scanning does. PET scanning is available in only a few specialist centres and its role in assessing and monitoring epilepsy has yet to be fully established: a special chemical, often mildly radioactive, is injected into the patient and its progress through and uptake by the brain is serially monitored. Developments of basic MRI scanning are also being developed for the same purpose and the next few years will bring exciting and useful developments.

## Prolactin blood level

A test that is of some use in investigating possible epilepsy is measuring, in a blood sample, taken 20 to 30 minutes after a seizure, the level of a hormone called prolactin (that 'lets down' milk into the breast after delivery of a child but which is present, in small amounts, in the blood of non-pregnant women and men). After a generalized tonic clonic or complex partial seizure there is, usually, a brief but dramatic rise in the blood level of this hormone in both men and women. This occurs after one seizure (but, if measured after a cluster of seizures, the reaction has usually exhausted and the blood level of the hormone may be misleadingly low). Since there are other causes for a raised prolactin level, there needs to be a comparison with a blood level of the hormone taken at the same time of day (or night) but not after a seizure in the same patient. False positive and false negative results of this test have been described, so on its own the test, though helpful, cannot be taken as completely conclusive.

## What about re-investigation?

This is a common question that patients ask (both 'why are you doing this again?' and 'isn't there some other test you can do?'). Both may be perfectly reasonable questions and require an answer. If the patient has been well investigated originally (good quality history, physical, and mental assessment, two EEGs (one sleep related) a 12-channel ECG, and a high power MRI) and a definitive diagnosis established then further investigation may well not be necessary. It may be done, however, because the original diagnosis was not a definitive one but made 'on the balance of probabilities' or the scan was not appropriate (CT instead of MRI) and it has been decided, since the patient is still having seizures, to investigate for surgery or to record a seizure on video EEG and ECG to clarify the diagnosis. Also, if much time has passed since the original diagnosis and investigation and the patient is still having seizures then a full re-appraisal can well be justified (particularly starting with the question 'is this really epilepsy that we are trying to treat?').

# 4

# So, if it isn't epilepsy then what is it?

## → Key points

- It can be difficult to correctly diagnose the cause of a seizure.
- Sometimes a spurious label of epilepsy is given to a seizure.
- Other physical causes of seizures can be mislabelled as epilepsy, as can emotional seizures.

There are many answers to the above question, which really lie outside the scope of this book (indeed would take a small textbook to answer). Both physical and emotional causes of non-epileptic seizures exist and both kinds can be mislabelled as epilepsy. What we can do is to give an example of each kind. The most important thing is that, if the patient's seizures turn out to be due to something other than epilepsy, they still need to be correctly diagnosed and appropriately managed and treated (and not just lobbed in the general direction of the local cardiologist or psychiatrist without a word of explanation to the patient). Often the patient gets blamed for what is, after all, the professional's mistake.

Evidence from specialist units suggests that sometimes up to 20% of people diagnosed elsewhere as having epilepsy don't actually have it when studied intensively (but some other condition instead mislabelled as epilepsy); one study indeed, from a very reputable epilepsy centre suggested that 50% of people admitted in 'status epilepticus' (see Chapter 5) to casualty departments didn't actually have epilepsy at all. Why is misdiagnosis so comparatively common?

Epilepsy is a diagnosis that can be made too quickly with too little thought or consideration for the many other causes of seizures or attacks and, once made and promulgated, can be a difficult diagnosis to change. So, possibly, if you have epilepsy it may be worth checking with your doctor how the diagnosis was actually made; occasionally you may decide, between you, to review all the evidence again and, if necessary, perhaps try to add to it.

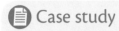 Case study

**Fiona** was 15 when her attacks first started. She would feel 'dizzy and out of this world' for a few seconds before falling to the floor unconscious, pale, and floppy; she would remain unconscious for about 30 seconds before recovering but remaining a little confused and pale for a few minutes longer. Over the years she had sustained several injuries (including a fractured wrist) in falling but had learnt to take notice of the 'aura' so that she was able to protect herself.

She had been investigated when the attacks first started. An EEG showed some right temporal theta activity (episodic slowing of the EEG rhythm recorded in the electrodes over the right temporal lobe) which was attributed to her epilepsy but a CT scan of her brain was normal. Over the years she had tried several different anticonvulsant drugs but only phenytoin had had any appreciable effect on the frequency of her seizures.

The seizures had had a severe effect on her life. She had finished education early and had had little employment since leaving school as the seizures frightened workmates considerably. Carol, a friend at work, had said, 'it's really scary; you look as though you are dead'. She did some voluntary work and lived quietly at home with her aging parents.

The account she gave of the attacks when first seen in a specialist epilepsy clinic aged 27 sounded more cardiovascular than epileptic and this was confirmed by a routine ECG performed at her first visit to the clinic which revealed a pathologically prolonged QT interval (part of the ECG signal) characteristic of the Romano–Ward syndrome (a rare serious disorder of the conducting mechanisms of the heart); curiously she had never had a previous ECG (phenytoin does have some therapeutic cardiovascular effects in its own right). The 'abnormality' in her first EEG, which had been ascribed to epilepsy, is actually not an abnormality at all in someone of 15; the team who saw her had been trying too hard to make the investigation 'fit' their diagnosis.

She was admitted to a cardiac unit that evening (since attacks can be fatal) and, after further tests, was fitted with a permanent cardiac pacemaker. She has had no further attacks and has withdrawn from the phenytoin. Currently she is employed and studying at night school, has a sexual partner, and is living apart from her parents.

# 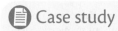 Case study

**Emily** was 36 and had had epilepsy for some 22 years. 'Can anything else be done for this tragic person?' her GP had asked when he referred her for further help. She had had her first seizure at 14, some 3 years after the start of her periods, when apparently asleep and alone in her bed at night; most of her subsequent seizures had also been nocturnal. She had had a variety of investigations over the years; several EEGs had shown bilateral theta activity particularly on over breathing (which had been interpreted as supporting a diagnosis of epilepsy but which actually does not, being quite normal in a person in their teenage years); two CT scans of her head some years apart had been reported as normal. Since she had moved frequently round the country it was difficult to keep track of all her investigations and treatments although several consultants had reviewed her over the years.

Her seizures were frequent, often several a week, although there had been times when she seemed to have been seizure-free for several months and her seizures were also much less frequent when she was menstruating. Her described night-time tonic clonic seizures were often prolonged and she had had several recent episodes of difficult-to-control 'status epilepticus'. She had recently moved back to the West Midlands to be near her ill and ageing mother with whom she had a difficult relationship. Emily's father had deserted the family when she was 11 and her mother had had a succession of usually short-term relationships with different men ever since. Life at home had been so chaotic that Emily had been briefly taken into care when she was 15.

At her initial appointment she unfortunately had a seizure in the corridor outside the consulting room before being able to give a history so that full assessment had to be curtailed and she was accordingly admitted for video EEG monitoring to get a better idea of the nature of her seizures.

Three things had been noted at her initial curtailed assessment: an EEG, taken about half an hour after the end of her seizure was normal, as was a serum prolactin level taken half an hour after the seizure started; blood levels of lamotrigine and phenytoin (the anticonvulsants she was currently being treated with) taken at the same time were both negative (suggesting that she had not taken either drug for some days at least).

During the video-EEG monitoring three seizures were recorded; one lasted several hours but the absence of any EEG change during the wild convulsive attack (similar to the other two shorter seizures with equal lack of EEG change) and the maintenance of normal oxygen levels throughout the prolonged seizure encouraged the hastily summoned consultant to merely wait and observe events. It was noticed that at the end of the attack she was crying.

It was clear that these were non-epileptic seizures and there was no evidence that she actually had epilepsy so her anticonvulsant medication was not restarted. It was obviously important to maintain contact with her; before leaving the unit she viewed the videotape of the seizures with the consultant and a nurse who had developed a good relationship with her. A great deal of discussion followed pointing out that even though her seizures were not those of epilepsy they were still real and important and with her help could be unravelled and controlled.

There followed, in regular sessions over about a year, a difficult exploration of her unhappy past; there was a history of sexual abuse from multiple perpetrators which took a long and fraught time to unravel and come to terms with, particularly as Emily began to realise that her mother knew about the abuse all the time but chose not to confront it (which was, indeed, the price the mother paid for male companionship).

Eventually the patient accepted that her mother was just as much a victim as she herself had been and her understandable anger subsided as did her seizures. The counselling was completed, the seizures have stopped; she is reconciled with her mother, is living with an understanding and supportive female partner, and is training to be a care assistant. It is likely that therapy was successful because she herself had decided that it was time to give up her seizures and 'get better' rather than run away again.

It is important to remember that women with actual epilepsy may also have suffered sexual abuse (which is not uncommon), so that a previous history of abuse does not mean that one is necessarily dealing with non-epileptic attacks.

# 5
# The risks of seizures

 Key points

- The risks associated with epilepsy can be reduced considerably by better treatment and sensible precautions.
- Precautions taken need to be geared to the patient and her particular seizures.
- All people with epilepsy need to adopt precautions when bathing or swimming.
- Injury in seizures is surprisingly common.
- Up to 1000 people in the UK die as the result of a seizure each year.
- Many of these deaths could be prevented.

There is no doubt that, overall, having epilepsy carries some risk to both life and limb; the risk is higher for some forms of epilepsy than others and least, of course, for those people with epilepsy whose seizures are perfectly controlled and without a cause, which itself carries some risk. This is something that may be, at some time, worth discussing with your specialist (who may, of course, want to talk it over with you—a survey carried out at a meeting of epilepsy specialists suggested that many would actually like to, but only do so, if the patient directly asks). What we are going to do is discuss some of the causes, where known, of the events that can, sadly, disrupt the life and existence of people with epilepsy. Obviously if the epilepsy is due to some condition like a malignant cerebral tumour or alcoholism then, even if perfectly controlled (sadly unlikely) one remains at risk from the causative condition itself.

## Risks depend on what happens in the seizure and where it occurs

- Is there loss of consciousness?
- Is there falling (sudden, stiff, or floppy)?

- Is there confused wandering?
- Is there a reliable warning? Is it long enough?
- Do seizures reliably take place in (say) bathroom, or at mealtimes?

---

## In a study of people with chronic epilepsy over 1 year:

- 10% had been to a casualty department as the result of seizure related injury.
- 50% were admitted overnight.
- Most had had a head injury and were often 'knocked out'.
- Head/facial cuts were common, as were cuts elsewhere.
- Wrist fractures were also common.
- Many women with epilepsy have softening of the bones due to their medication. They need to ensure they are taking enough calcium (see Chapter 17).

---

This means, if you continue to have seizures that you should stop and think about whether you can lessen the risk of injury by adopting some simple precautions:

- If you have a reliable warning that a seizure is coming do you bash on regardless hoping it won't happen this time (because sometimes it doesn't) or do you stop and put yourself in a safe recovery position?
- If you regularly have seizures in the early morning would it be better to bath or shower in the evening?
- If your child has atonic or tonic seizures should she wear a crash helmet to prevent recurrent damage to the head? Wearing a properly fitted and designed helmet can literally be life saving.

But, and this is an important 'but', some of you may well feel in the next few pages that we are being too 'namby-pamby', too overcautious; Harriet, as far as herself is concerned, certainly thinks so. So we offer the following precautions as suggestions that some of you may choose to follow because of the kind of seizure that you have. Risk taking is an essential part of growing up, but there are acceptable risks and extremely foolish ones; only you can decide. A properly safety-trained person watching over you may make you feel more secure and therefore have fewer seizures (this certainly applies if you have a Seizure Alert Dog®). On the other hand you may feel insufferably cosseted and over protected; it is really up to you.

# Precautions

## Eating

- If you regularly have seizures whilst eating (some people do) then try not to eat alone.
- Don't put too much in your mouth at once.
- Cut your food up small.
- Chew it carefully.
- Swallow it before taking the next mouthful.
- Make sure your companion knows how to do the 'Heimlich manoeuvre'.

## Travelling

- Cross the road on a pedestrian crossing whenever you can.
- Stand well back on the platform at railway stations.
- If possible, when out, have someone with you who can deal with a seizure.
- If you can't drive you may be entitled to free public transport (ask your doctor).

## The home

- It may be possible to have a companion if you are alone.
- If you live alone and have frequent night-time attacks assistance may be possible.
- If you sleep alone but with someone in the house get a competent automatic alarm.
- Use children's safety pillows at night.
- If you sleep with someone make sure they know appropriate first aid.
- Make your kitchen (and rest of the house) as safe as possible (see Chapter 16)—this particularly applies to mounting or descending stairs and cooking.

## Swimming

- Know how to swim—but don't swim on your own.
- Have a companion who knows what to do and who will watch you closely.
- In the sea stay in your depth.

- In the sea don't stay in too long (it's cold in the UK, even in summer).

- In a swimming pool always tell the attendant before you get in (wear a distinctive cap).

If you have a seizure in the pool:

- Your companion should support your mouth and nose clear of the water.

- S/he should then help you out when you have recovered—lifting a wet slippery person onto dry land whilst convulsing is too difficult.

- Practise first aid in the water with your companion.

- Suggest your companion has some time in the water on her or his own in recompense.

## Bathing or showering

- Fill the bath, adjust the temperature, and turn off the taps before you get in.

- If on your own not more than 4 inches (approximately 10 cm) of water and don't stay in long.

- Sit at the end away from the taps.

Try to have a companion (who knows first aid) either:

- In the bath if big enough (what fun!).

- In the bathroom.

- Just outside (in which case talk, as drowning is silent).

If showering:

- Make sure it is properly fitted with room to fall safely.

- Install an automatic water cut-off.

- Adjust the temperature before you get in.

- Have a companion if possible.

- Bath or shower at a time of day when you are least likely to have a seizure.

From an early age children can be taught to stay calm if a parent has a seizure (particularly if the rest of the family remain calm and clearly know what to do) and from about the age of 5 can be trained in the elementary first aid needed. 'I don't know what you said to him' one mother said to Tim about her 6-year-old child to whom Tim had talked about what to do if mother should have a seizure 'but apparently when I had one of my attacks in the supermarket recently he put me in the recovery position and then, sitting by my side, said loudly to the assembling shoppers 'bugger off—I'm in charge' and do you know, they did. I was proud of him'. Interestingly she has not had a seizure whilst shopping since, but now enters supermarkets with a broad smile as she remembers what her son said.

## Carry identification in an easily 'findable' place

- Your name and address.
- The name of someone to contact.
- Your GP's name, address, and phone number (and hospital clinic).
- Brief details of what usually happens in your seizure.
- How long it usually lasts for (and what to do if it doesn't stop).
- How soon you are likely to be fit (an interesting double meaning!) to go home.
- What first aid you will need, e.g. 'Guard my head whilst I am fitting; when the seizure is over roll me into the recovery position and lift my chin, make sure I am breathing properly and wait until I am fully awake; this usually takes about 5 minutes.'

## Sudden death in epilepsy (SUDEP)

Now we come to an important topic often not covered in books for people with epilepsy nor, indeed, sometimes in books for professionals, but which we feel has to be aired and discussed. We are talking about SUDEP. As already discussed, a seizure in the wrong place at the wrong time can lead to injury or even accidental death (e.g. falling downstairs, in the bath or crossing the road) but for most the risk can be markedly reduced by taking reasonable precautions. But some people with epilepsy die in, or shortly after, a seizure for no apparent reason. Since this usually happens when they are on their own it is difficult to be certain what the cause is. A recent British study has suggested that up to 1000 people a year with epilepsy die as a direct result of a seizure in the UK (proportionally more than die of asthma each year) and that many of these deaths could have been prevented by better treatment of people still having seizures.

The study suggested that it is a person's second seizure which is most likely to lead to SUDEP, so that most people have passed the maximum danger point in their epileptic career before they even realise they have epilepsy. This may, of course, be an argument for treating the first seizure if it recognized for what it is (see Chapter 6). Annie, whose sad case is described at the end of this chapter, died suddenly after a seizure and, although she had had a long period without seizures, when the seizures returned it was the second seizure that led to her unfortunate death. Her case illustrates the emotional stress that SUDEP places on both the family and the professionals and how they are often unable to support each other.

### Those most at risk

- People with tonic clonic and complex partial seizures.
- Those living alone.
- Aged between 20–40 years.
- People who have seizures in their sleep.
- Those possibly inconsistent in taking medication.

SUDEP after a seizure may initially be a respiratory rather than a cardiac arrest—so that cardiac massage alone (which has recently been advocated for immediate first aid in those who have suffered a cardiac arrest) may not be enough in the case of SUDEP and we would strongly advocate respiratory resuscitation as well.

### What can be done?

The survey previously mentioned certainly suggested that many of the deaths could have been prevented by the availability of better treatment. Many of the patients whose deaths were reviewed could have become seizure-free with more or better care. A change in attitude may be helpful, teaching both doctors and patients to better recognize that people with epilepsy don't necessarily need to have seizures and that, if the patient is still having them every effort should be made to control them. In those patients whose seizures cannot be controlled by medicine or surgery, thought should be given to teaching those who care for or live with the individual good quality first aid with sufficient practise to ensure that a clear airway is maintained and that the patient is put on her side immediately after a seizure.

## Suicide and epilepsy

Another sad reflection about the realities of having epilepsy is that the actual (the technical word is completed) suicide rate of people with epilepsy (particularly temporal lobe epilepsy) is higher than in the general population at large. There may be several reasons for this. Firstly, the life of someone with epilepsy may be overly stressful, with unnecessary barriers placed in the way of relationships and jobs, so that the individual feels lonely, useless, or unwanted. Secondly, people with epilepsy (particularly temporal lobe epilepsy) are subject to sudden and intense (but, luckily, usually short-lived) episodes of clinical depression in which determined suicide attempts may occur—for understandable and not always preventable reasons. Depressive episodes often occur at the point when medication has finally suppressed the seizures. In defence of doctors it should be pointed out that there is a kind of inverse relationship between seizures and depressive illnesses: indeed artificially induced and controlled seizures (electro-convulsive therapy) are still used effectively to swiftly relieve severe depression (and thus save life). Thirdly, of course, the person with epilepsy has in her or his possession medication for the epilepsy, which may be, if taken in overdose, a powerful poison.

# Serial and status epilepticus

Finally we need to consider serial epilepsy (when seizure rapidly follows seizure with some return of consciousness in-between) and status epilepticus (when seizure closely follows seizure without any intervening return of consciousness). Of the two, status is the more serious and the more common though both are a medical emergency and need to be brought under control as quickly as possible. Status occurs for a variety of reasons; recurrent tonic clonic seizures are the commonest (and most dangerous) although partial status also occurs and may be (since it often presents as prolonged clouded consciousness) difficult to recognize and easy to misinterpret as something else.

## Rectal diazepam

Status may sometimes be the presenting feature of epilepsy, particularly frontal seizures (see the Case study of Geraldine, Chapter 1) and may be a recurrent problem in some difficult-to-control epilepsies particularly associated with learning difficulty. In such cases teaching family or carers how to use emergency treatment such as rectal diazepam (e.g. Stesolid®) may be invaluable in cutting the status short (although the patient will still need to attend hospital, particularly because enough diazepam may have been given to render the patient unconscious and its controlling effect may wear off fairly quickly—the amount already given should be carefully recorded). Status may also occur in some people with epilepsy who suddenly discontinue their medication (either by accident or design) and drug withdrawal should always be undertaken slowly (even if the treatment appears to be totally ineffective) except in emergency when the anticonvulsant is doing something serious like causing aplastic anaemia (when its immediate withdrawal needs to be covered by some other rapidly acting drug).

## Status is dangerous—treat quickly and effectively

Frequent repetitive seizures and the lack of oxygen that often goes with them can have serious damaging effects on brain structure and function—indeed, generalized status, particularly if it is not brought under control quickly, carries a risk of being fatal. A patient in status needs admission to an Intensive Treatment Unit, prompt treatment, and specialist neurological care with EEG monitoring—this, in the UK, may be difficult to obtain. Intravenous diazepam or phenytoin remain the initial treatments, although newer and less toxic ones are being developed and it may be sometimes necessary to intubate, paralyse, and anaesthetize the patient for a while (this does need a specialist unit). When the status is under control some effort must be made to determine why it occurred and to try to prevent it from happening again.

## Pseudo-status

Some status turns out to be non-epileptic (which is one of the reasons why EEG monitoring is so necessary). Tim can remember one lady admitted to numerous hospitals by air ambulance from various remote parts of the country in 'severe status' who had never had a real seizure in her life; her ability to keep fitting (and smiling) despite vast amounts of intravenous diazepam was truly amazing. After much counselling the episodes have finally stopped.

So ends a chapter which at times must have read like an account of one unmitigated disaster after the other; do remember that most people with epilepsy have a few seizures, have them properly investigated (without a cause being found) and properly and promptly treated (with due attention being paid to their sex and childbearing needs), never have another seizure and, in the fullness of time, withdraw safely from their medication and go on living an uninterrupted life. It is important to remember that. In the next chapter we will start to consider how epilepsy should be treated.

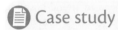 Case study

**Annie** was a shop assistant, 47, when first seen in an emergency epilepsy clinic. From the ages of 24 to 36 she had had complex partial seizures (loss of awareness, falling if standing, with lip smacking and chewing with occasional secondary generalization into a tonic clonic seizure) that were left temporal in origin on good EEG evidence; a CT scan was reported as normal. The attacks had stopped shortly after the birth of her second and last child but she continued to take phenytoin. She had entered the menopause about a year before the appointment. She was not taking hormone replacement therapy.

A week before being seen in the clinic she had had an unexpected complex partial seizure of the kind she had previously had; this was a disturbing reminder of an epilepsy that she had thought was behind her and she was understandably upset.

Physical examination was normal, as was an EEG and ECG; blood was taken for various investigations and an urgent sleep-deprived EEG and MRI were arranged for a few days later.

On the way home from the appointment she had a tonic clonic seizure in the car which her husband was driving. By the time he was able to draw into the side of the road and stop the car to attend to her the seizure was over; but she failed to start breathing again and, despite his frantic efforts, she was dead. Post-mortem examination showed no abnormality to account for her death. Clearly, however, this was a sudden death in epilepsy.

Naturally her husband and children were devastated by this terrible and completely unexpected event. No matter how blameless both professionals and relatives are it is impossible not to feel guilt when such a tragic event occurs. These feelings often drive both parties apart when they actually need to support each other but yet cannot because of their emotional reaction to the event. The husband, in particular, felt ashamed and guilty that he had not 'brought her round' and understandably projected much of this onto the clinic. He was put in touch with an organization that supplies information and support in such sad circumstances ('Epilepsy Bereaved') but he then broke contact and it is not known if he used their services or not.

# 6

# The management of epilepsy

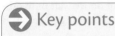 Key points

- What treatment shall we choose—almost invariably anticonvulsant drugs to start.
- When shall we start (first seizure or wait until epilepsy has settled in)? There are compelling arguments on both sides.
- For women, some commonly used drugs are best avoided.
- New drugs are expensive—but may have advantages for women.

## Advantage of treating first seizure

- More likely than not that there will be subsequent seizures eventually.
- Treatment can start slowly (less chance of side effects).
- Preventing the second seizure may prevent some SUDEP (see Chapter 5).
- Recent trial showed short-term gains in treating first seizure.
- If using lamotrigine or carbamazepine blood level indicates when enough given.
- Epilepsy is a distressing condition—the sooner it is treated and controlled the better.

## Advantage of treating second (or subsequent) seizures

- Not everyone will have a second seizure so unnecessary side effects avoided.

- Delaying does not alter outcome of treatment (equally likely to be successful).
- Short-term gains of treating first seizure are transient.
- Often the supposed first seizure turns out not to be the first one after all.

The treatment of epilepsy is, at the moment, mainly with medication. The first question is when shall we start? Do we treat the first seizure that occurs (assuming it really is the first seizure that we are dealing with) or do we wait until others have occurred and it is clear that the person we are helping is going to continue having seizures unless we try to stop them?

In the UK it is rare for the patient with new-onset epilepsy to be seen in a specialist clinic before he or she has had several seizures unless a rapid response clinic is established, open to GPs to refer to swiftly. Experience of one such clinic in Birmingham suggested that for every patient with epilepsy seen there was at least one other patient reviewed who had a condition resembling epilepsy but which was not the condition itself and who therefore needed different management. In a surprisingly high proportion of patients it was impossible to say what kind of attack had occurred and one had to wait for a second attack to be certain what one was dealing with (and, more often than initially expected, that second attack never came).

Moving the burden of diagnosis from the GP (who might see one new case every 2 years or so) to a clinic swiftly seeing several new patients a week was a distinct advantage, sharpened up clinical skills, and enabled the team to learn a lot. Swift intervention and assessment by an experienced clinical team reduced patient anxiety considerably. It also meant that the clinic rather than the GP was in charge of deciding both on diagnosis and on the most appropriate medication for the seizures, particularly important in women.

In many patients it is clear that the seizure presenting for assessment is not actually the first seizure; there have been unrecognized others beforehand. This is common in adolescents with juvenile myoclonic epilepsy presenting with their first tonic clonic seizure in whom it is swiftly apparent that there have been unrecognized myoclonic jerks for some time beforehand; likewise women presenting with their first tonic clonic seizure in pregnancy usually had a history of simple or complex partial seizures antedating the pregnancy but not recognized for what they were.

## Did the Birmingham clinic treat the first seizure or not?

### Yes, if (for example):

- The patient wanted it, after discussion (driving licence important, for example).
- First partial seizure with structural lesion on MRI (like hippocampal sclerosis).
- Primary generalized epilepsy with much epileptic activity in EEG.

### No, if (for example):

- The patient, after discussion, preferred not to start.
- The seizure was situational and related to circumstances that could be altered.
- Like, for instance, a sleepless, hung over, drugged, adolescent at a pop concert.

## What medication should be chosen?

In British men the decision is usually easy, in line with guidelines recently laid down by the National Institute for Health and Clinical Excellence (NICE) a body charged with examining the cost effectiveness of new drugs and deciding whether they can be prescribed on the British National Health Service and, if so, under what circumstances. The reason for following the guidelines is simple; new drugs, expensive to develop and test, cost much more than older drugs and may be no more effective (though possibly lacking some of the older drugs' unpleasant side effects). But, and this is an important but, women with epilepsy are not men with epilepsy writ small; they have periods, become pregnant, and hit the menopause; they need medication that, as far as possible, does not affect their ability to menstruate, conceive, use effective contraception, or bear healthy children. The choice of appropriate anticonvulsant medication for women with epilepsy is therefore sometimes different than that for men with epilepsy, a point that NICE does not completely recognize (although its recent epilepsy guidelines do give sufficient discretion for the clinician to make an informed choice as to the best anticonvulsant drug to use in a woman patient if she or he chooses to).

The first anticonvulsant tried is the one most likely to succeed, so in women it must be chosen carefully as it may be taken into the reproductive years and beyond. Points that need to be considered are:

- Some anticonvulsants impair calcium metabolism in later life.
- Find out what is known about risk to the baby in the womb and to fertility and periods.

◆ Avoid 'enzyme-inducing' drugs (see below) if possible in women taking 'the pill'.

◆ No drug is completely safe in pregnancy, but some are much riskier than others. Some drugs are known to affect fertility and/or menstruation—see Appendix 1.

So, the first drug is chosen; one usually starts with a low dose and slowly escalates it until the seizures stop. A low initial starting dose and slow escalation means that side effects are minimized and the patient does not need to take more of the drug than she needs. Some drugs, in addition to being enzyme-inducing to other liver metabolized drugs (speed up their breakdown in the liver), are 'auto-inducing'—in other words the initially achieved blood level then falls as the drug's metabolism gets to work so that a subsequent increase in dose may be needed to keep the patient seizure free; this is particularly important with carbamazepine. With some drugs (like lamotrigine and carbamazepine) a low, slow-dose regimen is particularly important to avoid potentially serious side effects (see individual drug accounts in Appendix 1).

# If seizure frequency is going up rapidly

One can take the risk of rapid escalation of the two drugs already mentioned (but if a serious reaction does occur then this is a potential disaster for the patient). So, it may be best to try drugs like levetiracetam, valproate, or phenytoin where a substantial and therapeutic dose can be given from the start (but valproate and phenytoin are both drugs with drawbacks as far as female patients are concerned—see later in this chapter).

If the first drug chosen, after being tried to the limits of tolerance (a medical term meaning until the side effects become impossible to bear, remembering that a doctor, who merely hears them described, can tolerate side effects much better than the patient who has to endure them) or taken to the extremes of conventional dosing, fails to control the seizures—then what?

## So, the first drug hasn't worked?

◆ An appropriate second drug is chosen and added in slowly.

◆ It should be appropriate and suitable, as far as possible, for the woman's special needs.

◆ If seizures stop (10% chance that they will) the first drug can be slowly withdrawn after a while.

◆ Some drugs are 'synergistic' (work better together than on their own) like valproate and lamotrigine (but the risk to babies' development is much increased).

## What if the second drug does not work?

Stop for a moment and reconsider:

◆ Is this really epilepsy we are trying to treat (consider re-investigation)?

◆ If it is, are we treating the right type (consider re-investigation)?

- Is there a cause we haven't recognized (like another drug you are taking)?
- If appropriate (e.g. one-sided temporal lobe epilepsy) consider surgery or consider vagal nerve stimulation or splitting the corpus callosum.
- Otherwise slow trawl through other suitable drugs (5% chance they will work).
- Removing one whilst adding one if possible.
- Remember doctors are much better at adding rather than subtracting drugs.
- Sometimes slow withdrawal down to just one drug works best (since drugs interact).
- Sometimes seizures can be modified (e.g. tonic clonic to simple partial).
- Sometimes behavioural, cognitive, or complementary treatments may be helpful.

## What about me?

One of the problems of epilepsy management (which we have heard many patients complain of) is that the patient herself seems left out of the loop; seizure control or lack of it seems to have nothing to do with her personally, but all to do with a little pill or a big operation: 'Isn't there anything I can do myself?' she wonders only to be told 'just keep on taking the tablets'. Yet epilepsy comes from the brain from which also derives our thoughts, feelings, and emotions—surely there must be some connection somewhere?

## How much do anticonvulsants differ from each other?

- Some drugs are almost certainly safer for women and their offspring.
- Some drugs are more powerful than others (but may have powerful side effects). It is difficult to tell, as new drugs are not usually tested against each other.

New anticonvulsants do cost considerably more than the older ones. Manufacturers, who may have spent several million pounds testing a drug in order to get it to market, once the drug is launched, have then only got 15 years to recoup their costs and make a profit to please their shareholders before other drug firms can launch their own brand of the drug without having had to do any of the prior research; and it is going to take doctors, who, rightly, are somewhat conservative in their prescribing—especially with epilepsy—a few years to learn how to best use the new compound.

Fifteen years or so after the launch of a drug onto the market several different brands of it may then exist which is why, when we list them, we will use the official (generic) names of the drugs rather than the trade name(s)—the 'official' name is, if you like, the proper name. It is worth checking with your doctor which you are taking: if, for instance, you are taking Lamictal® (the original brand of lamotrigine) and you are seizure free, it is worth sticking with it since if you switched to another brand of the drug you run the risk of having seizures again. Although this is not very likely to happen it has been known to, unfortunately. This is because manufacturers of the other brands of the same drug are allowed a little latitude in the same dose of the drug reaching the same blood level. Now with some drugs a 10% difference in blood level between two versions of the same drug does not matter very much; but with anticonvulsants it can sometimes be important and can mean loss of efficacy (as with lamotrigine) or intoxication (as with phenytoin). If you are already taking an alternative try to stick to the same brand, which will need your doctor's co-operation since she or he will have to specify it on your prescription.

If two anticonvulsant drugs were equally effective and equally safe but one was much more expensive than the other, doctors would obviously use the cheaper one. But if the more expensive one doesn't disrupt the periods or cause a significant risk of fetal abnormality then obviously they would use it for their female patients. The doctor's first duty is to her or his patient, not to the government.

## What is a 'half-life'?

This refers to the time taken for the blood level of a drug to fall to half its peak level (this peak level is usually achieved within 2 hours after ingestion and maintained for a varying length of time). The efficacy of the drug is reduced when the blood level falls below the half-life blood level; some drugs like carbamazepine have a comparatively short half-life so may need to be taken 3 or 4 times a day to maintain an effective blood level (but see the 'retard' formulation in Appendix 1).

## Side effects

Do remember that most serious side effects (like hypersensitivity reactions) are rare and a prescribing doctor should be alert to them; they are a potential risk for all drugs, even the humble aspirin. It may take some time for a serious side effect to appear, be recognized, and acted upon. We often know far more about the drawbacks of the older drugs than we do of the newer ones. Do remember that although we have tried to make the information in Chapter 7 as accurate as possible for early in 2008, views may well change and, as always, you will need to discuss the most accurate and up-to-date information with your medical or nursing adviser.

# Finally, a word of warning

If you have, or have had, epilepsy then on no account take any benzodiazepine drug (like diazepam) as a tranquillizer because of the risk of inducing seizures when you withdraw from it (they also have a marked 'normalizing' effect on the EEG which can be misleading). There is no problem if you are taking them for epilepsy itself (see clobazam and clonazepam—and the correct use of diazepam—in Appendix 1) because when the time comes to withdraw you will come off them slowly and will only have taken diazepam as a single-dose rescue remedy.

# 7

# The drugs in use— pros and cons

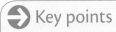 Key points

- There are a number of drugs available for epilepsy in the UK.
- Some are obsolete or are potentially dangerous; we tell you in case you don't know.
- Some cause problems relating to menstruation, fertility, child development, and the menopause.
- Every woman with epilepsy should take folic acid 5 milligrams daily from before she becomes pregnant and all the way through her pregnancy (or at least the first 4 months).
- Women taking certain drugs should take vitamin K from the 36th week (listed).

If you are a woman who may become pregnant it is important to know of any possible consequences if you are taking a particular drug. If you are prescribed a new drug it is a good idea to discuss possible side effects with the person giving it to you and if she or he is not familiar with them then it should be looked up in the *British National Formulary* (*BNF*), a new edition of which is published twice a year (other countries have similar authoritative publications). If you are taking other medication not related to your epilepsy (an oral contraceptive, for instance) it is particularly important that the person prescribing the drug checks the section on drug interactions. Information about and knowledge of drugs can change rapidly so always make sure an up-to-date edition is consulted.

Information in this chapter has been checked against the Spring 2008 edition of the *BNF*, although, since it is an 'official' publication it has to be completely sure of its facts, whereas we can sometimes express an opinion based on our own particular experience which may be at variance with the 'official' position. For example the *BNF* states, quite correctly, that there is a potential risk to the developing baby from all anticonvulsant drugs. This is true but equally evidence is accumulating that the risk is almost certainly higher with some drugs than others and that some are better avoided by the potentially pregnant woman if possible. Obviously it would be best if the woman could completely withdraw from all anticonvulsant drugs before she becomes pregnant (see Chapter 14) but for many women this is just not possible (since uncontrolled epilepsy is dangerous for both mother and child) and she and her medical advisor have to make an individual decision about the best course to take based on her particular circumstances and on what evidence is available, fragmentary and incomplete as that may be.

## Side effects

We have classified side effects in Appendix 1 as follows:

- Whether a drug is enzyme inducing or not (and by how much)—such a drug enhances the activity of liver enzymes that break down other liver metabolized drugs (like 'the pill' and some other anticonvulsants) so that their blood level is reduced.
- Dose-related—the bigger the dose the more likely the side effect and dose reduction may remove it.
- Hypersensitivity—even a small dose in a predisposed individual may produce an often potentially serious side effect to which most patients are immune.
- Chronic toxicity—caused by long-term use of the drug.
- Those related to pregnancy and breast feeding—where known.
- Do remember that information may change as further experience is gained and other studies are completed
- Always discuss these issues with your medical and nursing advisor for up-to-date advice; this is particularly important if you have other medical conditions like chronic liver or renal disease or suffer from something like porphyria.

Complete lists of possible side effects for each drug might well occupy several pages so we have only included the more serious and well attested ones. All drugs, for instance, can make some people feel dizzy, headachy, tired and/or confused so we have not listed these. It is important if you start any new anticonvulsant drug that you are alert to any new side effects and, in particular, if you suddenly develop fever, mouth ulcers, sore throat, bruising, rash, or unexplained bleeding that you let your doctor know at once, as these symptoms may presage something serious (but, of course, may not).

First we deal with two drugs that are not anticonvulsants but essential vitamins for the woman with epilepsy.

# Folic acid

This is a vitamin with some similarities to vitamin B12 in that it is essential for the proper formation of red blood cells so that deficiency of it leads to an unpleasant form of anaemia and deficiency of it in early pregnancy can lead to a serious disorder of the lower spinal cord in the baby (spina bifida).

◆ All women should take 400 micrograms of folic acid daily from before they intend to become pregnant; there is good trial evidence that this protects against spina bifida.

◆ Women who have already had a child with spina bifida should take 5 milligrams of folic acid daily from before they become pregnant: again there is good trial evidence that this is protective against a recurrence. 400-microgram tablets can be bought over the counter; 5-milligram ones have to be prescribed.

◆ Women with epilepsy are more at risk of having a child with spina bifida than women who do not have epilepsy, particularly if they are taking certain anticonvulsants; they should therefore also take 5 milligrams of folic acid from before they start trying to become pregnant (a recent report suggested for a year before). With some anticonvulsants (see individual descriptions later) folic acid should continue to be taken throughout the pregnancy; with other anticonvulsants some authorities suggest stopping taking folic acid after 4 months of the pregnancy, although other authorities suggest continuing (and, indeed, continuing after the birth if another pregnancy is a possibility).

Before you start folic acid your doctor should check that your blood level of vitamin B12 is normal. Once your childbearing days are over then discontinue folic acid as there is some evidence that continuing to take it in middle age and beyond may lead to health problems (although with certain anticonvulsants (now obsolete, see later in this chapter) you will need to continue to take folic acid supplements. There are rumours that British bread is about to be fortified with folic acid (in Canada it already is with a resultant significant reduction in the number of babies born with spina bifida) but you will still need to take folic acid before and during pregnancy if you have epilepsy.

# Vitamin K

The infants of all women are given 1 milligram of this vitamin at birth to prevent a serious blood disorder which otherwise can occur at this time—haemorrhagic disease of the newborn. Mothers taking an enzyme-inducing anticonvulsant (carbamazepine, oxcarbazepine, phenobarbital, primidone, phenytoin, topiramate, and zonisamide) should take 10 milligrams of the vitamin by mouth daily from the 36th week of the pregnancy until birth (and their child should also have the injection) as these drugs are known to partially interfere with the absorption of the vitamin from the gut and there is some evidence that taking this otherwise harmless vitamin does protect the child from the disorder.

- *First-line drugs* are those that can be prescribed as the first anticonvulsant to be tried.
- (Caution with carbamazepine and oxcarbazepine in those taking other drugs.)
- *Second-line drugs* are good second choices (as are previously unused first-line drugs).
- *Third-line drugs* should be used if the first two fail. Topiramate and valproate are best avoided in women who may become pregnant. This is not always possible and they are first-line in all other patients.
- *Special use drugs* are used in particular forms of epilepsy (like pre-menstrual).
- *Obsolete drugs* are best avoided or withdrawn from except in special circumstances.

**Table 7.1** Anticonvulsant drugs for women before the menopause

| First line | Second line | Third line | Special use | Obsolete |
|---|---|---|---|---|
| Carbamazepine | Gabapentin | Clobazam | Acetazolamide | Ethosuximide |
| Lamotrigine | Pregabalin | Clonazepam | Clobazam | Phenobarbital |
| Levetiracetam | Tiagabine | Lacosamide | Diazepam | Phenytoin |
| Oxcarbazepine | | Topiramate | Rufinamide | Primidone |
| | | Valproate | | Vigabatrin |
| | | Zonisamide | | |

**Table 7.2** Anticonvulsant drugs for women after the menopause

| First line | Second line | Third line | Special use | Obsolete |
|---|---|---|---|---|
| Carbamazepine | Gabapentin | Clobazam | Diazepam | Ethosuximide |
| Lamotrigine | Pregabalin | Clonazepam | | Phenobarbital |
| Levetiracetam | Tiagabine | Lacosamide | | Phenytoin |
| Oxcarbazepine | | Zonisamide | | Primidone |
| Topiramate | | | | Vigabatrin |
| Valproate | | | | |

Valproate and topiramate now become first-line; still avoid phenobarbital and phenytoin if at all possible because of their metabolic effects, particularly in the menopause. A full list of the available drugs is in Appendix 1.

## When can anticonvulsants be withdrawn?

This is an interesting question the answer to which depends on the individual, the type of epilepsy she or he has, and its cause (where known). This is a particularly important question for the woman with epilepsy planning pregnancy to try to answer (even if she occasionally gets a rather dusty response). It is complicated by the need to remain seizure free if one has a valid driving licence and decision-making is made more difficult by the fact that although it is probably best for the child if the mother was not taking an anticonvulsant, at least in the early stages of pregnancy, seizures in pregnancy are potentially dangerous for both mother and child and are therefore best avoided. It becomes very much an individual decision as it is indeed for children with epilepsy who are seizure free. A fuller discussion takes place in Chapter 13, Preconception counselling.

## Diary keeping—pros and cons

Some people with epilepsy keep diaries of their seizures—sometimes for many years with the view that there may be some pattern to them that time will eventually reveal—'look at that,' as one Scotsman excitedly said to Tim whilst exhibiting a diary that stretched back over many years 'I tell ye mon it's the porridge for sure.' Looking at his reddened nose and face Tim thought it might be the potage rather than the porridge that caused the seizures but loyally said (as one Scotsman to another) 'well if you are so sure why not try something else for breakfast?,' only to be told with scorn 'but I like my fxxxxxx porridge!'

Others do not keep a diary in the sometimes mistaken belief that there is no pattern to their seizures. It is, however, sometimes a useful thing to do particularly for a few months at the start of the illness or during changes in treatment making sure, if you do so, that you record more than a laconic 'had seizure today' but rather also note what was happening before the attack (one patient who did this for a few months realised that it only happened when her mother-in-law came for the day – see Case study, Jane, in Chapter 8) and, if you are a woman, where you are in your menstrual cycle accurately (as studies have shown that many more women feel they have premenstrual seizures than is actually the case). So, at least for a while, a diary of seizures, particularly if it records other events and times, can be useful and worth doing but should not become an obsession; this is something worth discussing with your health professional.

## Breastfeeding and epilepsy

There is no doubt that breastfeeding helps to bind mother and child closer together and provides the child with specifically designed nutrition during the early post-natal months. But breastfeeding can be exhausting as the child may need feeding every 2–3 hours and certainly during the night, interfering with sleep (and possibly, therefore, making seizures more likely). Also some of the mother's medication will get into the breast milk (the amount varies depending on the drug involved) so the child will be ingesting unneeded and possibly harmful anticonvulsant at a time when its developing metabolism may be unable to cope with the drug load; this is particularly the case if the child is premature. It is true that the child has been exposed to the drug for the 9 months it has been in the womb but during that time, of course, the mother's metabolism was protecting the child; now, it is on its own. So what should be done? Should the woman breastfeed or not, bearing in mind that drug manufacturers generally advise not to? (Their information leaflet should accompany each prescription.) If she doesn't breastfeed at all the child is suddenly withdrawn from a drug it has become accustomed to over the previous 9 months and may possibly have withdrawal symptoms (Tim has certainly seen babies 'jittery' for a few days after being born to mothers taking phenobarbital and not breastfed).

What we have done is indicate, for each drug in Appendix 1, whether the evidence is that breastfeeding should be avoided completely, whether it perhaps should be confined to the first 4 or 5 days so that the child is not suddenly deprived of the anticonvulsant but that further feeding after that point is not advised (often to prevent a too sleepy baby or because the drug manufacturers strongly advise against it), where (in Tim's experience) breastfeeding appears to be safe, and finally when we don't know. This latter advice applies only to babies born at term; if they are born prematurely then caution is advised (and if the mother is taking lamotrigine (which, at term, is safe) she should avoid breastfeeding altogether if the child is premature). This is something you must discuss with your medical or nursing advisor. Do remember that the milk that comes down into the breast in the first few days after birth, the colostrum, is not quite the same as later breast milk.

## Expressing breast milk

Breastfeeding is tiring and you need your sleep; why not express your breast milk into bottles, so that your partner does the night feeds; your midwife will advise you about breast pumps. If you are taking a drug that precludes breastfeeding and you particularly want to give the child some breast milk then banks of breast milk are available obtained from mothers that have more than enough; discuss this with your midwife. Remember that breastfeeding, until you are used to it, is often extremely hard work (and still hard work after you are used to it, although very rewarding) and you will need practical advice and support to achieve it particularly as this hard work comes at a time when most mothers are a little out of sorts and miserable; this is quite normal, does not last long and is no more likely if you have epilepsy than if you don't.

## Make yourself safe

If you have epilepsy it is probably best not to breastfeed completely on your own if you can arrange this and to ensure that when you do it you are in a position where, if you did have a seizure, the baby will not come to harm—for example, sitting on the floor with your back supported. This again is something to discuss with your midwife because the advice that you need will depend upon the kind of seizure that you have, but in the first few weeks after birth you must assume that because of fatigue and tiredness and the physiological changes that take place in the body after birth (the puerperium as medics call it) seizures are more likely unless you can get proper rest, which is why having a supportive partner is so important (or a good, sustainable, long-lasting support network). So, look up your drug(s) above and in Appendix 1, see what we suggest (as always do remember that advice may change as more research is done and, if you are taking two drugs the risk to your baby may be greater) and then discuss it with your physician or specialist nurse and your midwife (you may, of course, need to educate her or him about epilepsy—why not lend them this book, or suggest it is bought?).

# 8

# Other treatments, other problems

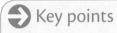 Key points

This section includes:

- Surgical treatment of epilepsy.
- Incidental (removal of brain lesion).
- Direct—removing surgical focus as in temporal lobe surgery.
- Palliative—as in hemispherectomy.
- Indirect—as in vagal nerve stimulation.
- Psychological treatments—behavioural and cognitive.
- Ketogenic diet treatment.
- Complementary and alternative therapies.
- Travelling abroad—health insurance, malarial prophylaxis etc.
- Having an anaesthetic if you have epilepsy.

## Surgical treatment of epilepsy

Although a layperson tends to regard brain surgery as inherently dangerous and disturbing, only to be carried out as a last resort in the clinically desperate, it actually has an essential place in the management of epilepsy and, in the UK at least, fewer people receive it for epilepsy than would undoubtedly benefit from it. There are four roles for surgery in helping to manage epilepsy:

- Surgical treatment of a brain lesion (like a tumour) causing seizures. Often if the lesion is removed the epilepsy will eventually resolve.
- Surgical treatment of epilepsy itself (e.g. unilateral temporal lobe epilepsy). 80% chance that seizures will disappear and medication withdrawn.
- Palliative surgery (e.g. hemispherectomy for unilateral motor seizures). Often epilepsy stops, rehabilitation can begin and hemiplegia no worse.

◆ Vagal nerve surgery (left vagal nerve stimulation device). A Birmingham study showed that 10% of patients become seizure free (mostly in partial onset epilepsy, but it can be used in other types).

Particularly in left temporal lobe surgery (and sometimes if the lesion is on the right, depending to some extent on whether the patient is right or left handed), the surgeon may want to carry out a 'Wada test' (another eponym of a justly famous neuroscientist). During this test one temporal lobe at a time is anaesthetized using a flexible tube inserted into the groin and run up the arterial system into the right or left carotid artery (in the neck) so that a soluble anaesthetic can be injected to temporarily switch off one half of the cortex so that the other half can be tested to ensure that it can function in the absence of the other one; not the most pleasant test in the world but sometimes essential.

Before surgery it is important to have an up-to-date, high-quality MRI and several seizures recorded on videotape and EEG to ensure that the epilepsy is actually coming from the part of the brain that the surgeon is proposing to remove. This is extremely important; just because you have a lesion in your brain it does not necessarily mean that it is causing your epilepsy and there have been one or two sad cases where operations were done for epilepsy on the brains of people who did not actually have it.

If you are a woman wanting children and are a potential candidate for surgery then it may be best to have the surgery before having children because if it is successful (and it usually is) it is often possible, after a year or two, to withdraw from medication.

### When should surgery be attempted?

This depends on both the epilepsy and its cause. For many people with epilepsy, failure of two first-line drug treatments of epilepsy should raise the possibility of surgery, as the chance of drug treatment being successful is then small: certainly, at least, assessment for surgical treatment can continue whilst a third drug is tried.

## Psychological treatments

In epilepsies that are resistant to drug treatment and unsuitable for surgery, psychological treatments have been tried, usually on an individual basis with few fully controlled trials (although surgical treatment has not often been tested in this way). There are problems in assessing the results of such treatments.

A behavioural approach to a person's seizures implies teaching the patient to recognize the cues that indicate that a seizure is about to start (or has already started) or is very likely to start and to respond to them by altering their behaviour rapidly, usually to decrease anxiety. Most people, understandably, faced with the imminent arrival of a seizure feel anxious and afraid; this emotional response, of course, actually makes the seizure more likely to occur and, even in people well used to their seizures, may become an automatic reaction that can actually increase seizure frequency particularly if coupled with fear of seizures in particular situations (see the case studies below). If one can teach the person to instantly and automatically relax when seizures are imminent (and to recognize when they are likely to occur) they can sometimes be averted. To do this usually requires several months of careful diary-keeping (to accurately identify seizure triggers and the individual's reaction to them) and to learn to relax or to recognize and prevent chains of negative thoughts (however understandable) that tend to be the automatic reaction to the threat of a seizure. This latter approach, which can also sometimes be successful, is cognitive therapy. Both approaches may require the help of a skilled therapist. Here are two examples.

 Case study

**Denise** was a specialist nurse who had, despite trying several different anticonvulsant drugs (and being unsuitable for surgery), occasional tonic clonic seizures in her sleep. Since they occurred only in her sleep she continued at work, but was often grumpy and sluggish at work in the daytime if she had had a seizure in the night and was therefore keen to see if anything else could be done for them (and, yes, she had had EEG monitoring and they were epileptic seizures). She kept a careful diary for a few months and it became clear that there were two factors in her life associated with her night-time seizures. The first was a row with her live-in and somewhat indolent boyfriend—the rows were frequent, although not always followed by a seizure; the second was related to working a late shift (2 pm to 10 pm) followed next day by an early shift (7 am to 3 pm). On such nights she found sleep difficult, as it was impossible to 'let go' of the day's events and stop thinking about them.

Joint counselling was suggested for the first factor, but she said 'don't worry, I've already got rid of the lazy bxxxxx and I feel much better for it—should have done it a long time ago!' Since she couldn't avoid an occasional 'double shift' without, as she saw it 'letting down my mates' she was taught a relaxation method to use on stressful nights to ensure rapid and restful sleep. Since ditching her boyfriend and learning to relax and sleep properly she has not had a seizure and has been able to simplify (but not totally withdraw from) her medication.

Case study

**Jane**, 26, had infrequent but distressing complex partial seizures involving a motionless stare followed by 30 seconds of incomprehensible and nonsensical speech originating (on EEG monitoring) in her left temporal lobe but without an MRI lesion and therefore surgery was thought inadvisable. What her seizure diary revealed was that seizures only occurred when her mother-in-law visited or a visit was imminent. The lady in question was overbearing and critical but Jane's husband felt obliged to continue to invite her to their home. Within a few hours of her appearance in the family home Jane would have a seizure and have to retire to bed for an hour or two to recover. Mother-in-law would often make things worse by enquiring loudly why her son had chosen to marry 'an epileptic' and whether he really wanted to risk having children with her.

Jane was therefore given a course of cognitive therapy, helping her to change her cycle of negative thinking about her mother-in-law to a more positive one, including associating her with a slightly salacious image of the mother-in-law standing, naked and terrified, in a field of curious, lowing, and butting bullocks, which she had once described as happening to herself on a camping trip. The seizures stopped, although to this day the mother-in-law is puzzled as to why she is now greeted by a smile from her daughter-in-law, who subsequently reduced her medication just to carbamazepine and has successfully had two children.

Although both patients became seizure free (both, wisely in our opinion, decided to stay on some medication) it cannot be proven that the behavioural or cognitive therapies they received actually caused them to become seizure free: in both cases the decision to make life-enhancing changes may have been equally important and to 'come to terms' with the epilepsy may have been even more so. We just don't know; but the feeling 'I am doing something for myself' may be of equal importance.

## Diet treatments and epilepsy

By and large if you have epilepsy you can make your culinary choices free of any fear that, however bizarre, what you eat may make your epilepsy worse. But there is good evidence that occasionally, particularly in otherwise difficult-to-treat children's epilepsy, a specific type of diet, the ketogenic diet, may be invaluable and can render such children seizure free. But only a few centres offer such treatment (your consultant should know which is your nearest one) and the diet means a lot of sustained cooking for the parents of often not very palatable food and needs the attention of a skilled dietician if it is going to work. The recent NICE guidelines suggest trying at least two first-line anticonvulsant drugs before attempting the diet and that would be right; but occasionally the diet if properly adhered to (and that is not easy) may render a child, with otherwise intractable seizures, totally seizure free.

## Non-medical (alternative or complementary) treatments

This is a topic that is prone to make physicians red with anger and write letters to *The Times* and mutter dismissively about unproven alternative treatments. Well, yes, and no. Most people with epilepsy will get seizure freedom and a normal life with conventional medical, surgical or, sometimes, psychological treatment and have no need to look elsewhere; but for some this is not the case and they may feel, as mentioned earlier, left out of the loop and merely passive recipients of medical or surgical care.

They may of course want to try a non-medical treatment for something else in their life which has apparently nothing to do with their epilepsy and, because they think their doctor is likely to be hostile, don't mention that they are now taking St. John's Wort from the local health food shop for their recurrent winter depression and wonder why their seizure frequency has gone up, not realising that the St. John's Wort (which is excellent for mild-to-moderate depression) has had an effect on the blood level of the carbamazepine they are also taking.

Non-medical treatment should be complementary to medical treatment, not alternative to it, if you have epilepsy and your medical advisor (even if she or he disagrees and thinks you are wasting your money) kept fully in the picture. So next time you want to try acupuncture for your bad back (for which it can be helpful—yes, there is good trial evidence) don't forget to tell your doctor; but don't think it will help your epilepsy (because there have been properly controlled trials to show that it doesn't). Make sure, too, that the acupuncturist knows about your epilepsy in case she or he has to modify their approach. There is some (admittedly uncontrolled) evidence that a few complementary non-medical treatments may be helpful for some people with epilepsy—hypnosis, formal relaxation training, massage, and aromatherapy—very much geared to the individual and the triggers of her or his particular epilepsy. So if you want to try a complementary therapy discuss it with your doctor and a reputable therapist first and then decide if you want to go ahead or not.

## Travelling abroad

It is worth reading this section even if you are only going abroad for a couple of weeks but it is becoming the fashion for people to spend time abroad, up to 12 months, as a 'gap year' before settling down to study or work. This has much to commend it, but what if the prospective traveller has epilepsy? Is it safe? The answer, taken both from Tim's experience as a medic and Harriet's as an inveterate traveller, is undoubtedly 'yes', providing certain common-sense precautions are taken (and we do mean common-sense).

If you are prone to seizures then travel with someone who knows what to do if you should have one; take a small supply of clobazam (for you to use), and possibly rectal diazepam (for your companion to use—make sure she or he knows how to), and on long flights across several time zones perhaps take 10 milligrams of clobazam on the flight and on your first night in the new environment to ensure sleep and the same on your return—but no more than this. Divide your medication into two lots so that you always have a couple of weeks or so of anticonvulsant with you in case the rest is locked in your case, which has flown to Australia whilst you are in Canada (it has happened).

Remember that your medication may not be available where you are going (or may be very expensive) so, if necessary, arrange with those at home and your GP to replenish your supply at a safe forwarding address and remember if you are going to a hot country that medication is best kept cool; in the country you are visiting it may have a different trade name which is why knowing the official (generic) name is so important. Try to arrange to take a letter with you from your clinic or GP saying what medication you are taking (this is important), what kind of epilepsy you have, and what investigations have been done. If possible an email address of your clinic at home will be useful in case medical authorities abroad want to get in touch.

Get health insurance if you can as medical care in some countries like the USA is very expensive (and the dear old US of A is the only country where some of Tim's patients had difficulties with the authorities about taking medication with them, even when it was not available there at the time). If you are liable to have seizures and are going to less developed parts of the world it will be worth checking what the local population think about and how they are likely to react to seizures and taking a letter with you about your medical history, translated into the local language (your local university may be helpful here). If you want to read of the experience of other people with epilepsy abroad then get hold of a copy of the paper referenced below.

Betts, T. (2004). Pre-departure counselling and an email contact service for patients with epilepsy faring abroad for long periods of time. *Seizure* **13**, 139–41.

And finally, sex and malaria, not necessarily in that order. Do use (or make sure your companion uses) reliable condoms—take some with you and take a small supply of the morning-after pill as well and know how and when to use it and whether you are taking anticonvulsant medication that means that you need to take more of the morning-after pill than usual; do remember that AIDS is prevalent in some parts of the world so always use condoms even if you are taking the pill. By all means enjoy yourself but be cautious and remember that 'the strongest oath is straw to the fire in the blood' and also dissolves in alcohol. Do remember that the standards of sexual behaviour that we regard as perfectly normal in this country, particularly if you are a woman, may be totally unacceptable in other countries—yes, we know, double standards, but some countries do have them plus rather punitive laws!

If you are going to a malarial area make sure you take the appropriate antimalarial drug from before you arrive until well after you leave (this is important so check carefully with your doctor how long this should be) and remember that the person you are seeking advice from should know that you have epilepsy, since some antimalarial drugs are potentially convulsant or you may have to take more than usual because of the anticonvulsant you are taking; you will need up-to-date advice for the area you are going to.

## Having an anaesthetic

A light brief anaesthetic should be no problem if you have epilepsy, although it is important that the anaesthetist and surgeon know of your epilepsy and your medication before the operation, particularly so that they can arrange the operation around the times you usually take your medication and the anaesthetist avoid any possible interactions between the drugs you are taking and the drugs she or he proposes to use. If you have a longer anaesthetic and a longer surgical procedure (particularly if you cannot take solids for some time after the operation) then thought will have to be given as to how best to continue your anticonvulsant medication; this will usually be in liquid form as syrup down your stomach tube (the Ryle's tube to give it its medical name), or sometimes via a drip into a vein, or even into your back passage (the French way). Sometimes a brief course of clobazam may also be used to give you even greater protection from a seizure which is best avoided if you are recovering from major surgery. If it is an emergency operation, then the best way of continuing your medication can be sorted out afterwards; it is useful, as we say elsewhere in this book, if you always carry with you a letter detailing information about your epilepsy and the medication you take for it and giving contact details for both your GP and specialist.

# Part 2

# 9

# Being a woman, having epilepsy

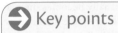 Key points

◆ Epilepsy can affect the timing and regularity of menstruation.

◆ The menstrual cycle can also have an effect on epilepsy; about 12% of women have seizures tightly linked to their menstrual cycle.

◆ The fertility of women with epilepsy is probably less than women in general.

◆ Up to 20% of women have more ovarian cysts (follicles) than thought usual, and this can be due to a condition called the polycystic ovary syndrome.

## An important general point

Let's start with an important warning; this section will only apply to some women, some of the time. Many women with epilepsy sail through their periods, their pregnancies, and their eventual menopause with no problems at all even if they are taking the medication that theoretically may not be the best for them. They are the lucky ones. Almost all women with epilepsy in the developed world take anticonvulsant medication so it is sometimes difficult to decide if it is the epilepsy itself or the medication being taken for the epilepsy that poses the potential problem.

## Epilepsy and the menstrual cycle

Epilepsy itself can affect the timing and regularity of the menstrual cycle and possibly fertility; to what extent is open to question. We know that after tonic clonic and complex partial seizures there is a measurable (and potentially diagnostic) release of the hormone prolactin; since this involves production in the pituitary gland and the hypothalamus other hormones and their precursors may be released as well which potentially can upset the delicate and interlocking mechanisms of the menstrual cycle. A recent and comprehensive study in the UK certainly suggested that the fertility of women with epilepsy is less than that of women who do not have epilepsy.

## What is the polycystic ovary syndrome (PCOS)?

A woman with a normal menstrual cycle sheds the lining of her womb (menstruates) roughly every 28 days. A new lining (the endometrium) then develops and grows ready to receive a fertilized egg (ovum): the ovum itself is released from one of the ovaries at about day 14 of the cycle. Several follicles (cysts) have begun to develop in the ovary towards becoming an ovum but most never get that far, die, and are reabsorbed back into the ovary. If the released ovum is not fertilized by a male sperm it dies and the endometrium is shed again; if it is fertilized then the endometrium develops further and eventually becomes the placenta that nourishes the fetus in the womb. In a normal ovary there are no more than 10 cysts visible at any one time in the various stages of development and decline; in a polycystic ovary there are more than 10. A woman with too many cysts in her ovary is said to have 'polycystic ovaries'. If, in addition, she has hormone changes (measured if possible between days 2–6 of the cycle when levels are normally at their lowest) of a raised follicle stimulating hormone (FSH), and/or a raised luteinizing hormone level (LH), and/or a raised testosterone hormone level then she is said to have PCOS, present in 4–5% of women and often, but not invariably, associated with overweight, irregular periods, and relative infertility.

A recent Birmingham study showed that women who had primary generalized epilepsy and who were taking and had only ever taken a single anticonvulsant (either sodium valproate, lamotrigine, or carbamazepine) were more likely to have polycystic ovaries than women of the same age who did not have epilepsy (the control group). But it was only the women taking sodium valproate and who were not taking 'the pill' (which is protective against the syndrome) that were significantly more likely to have PCOS when the hormone level tests for this condition were measured. It is important to emphasise that not every woman taking sodium valproate is going to develop PCOS; other factors are involved. But it is one of the reasons why women of childbearing age should avoid this drug if possible.

PCOS was first described in the late 1930s in a group of American women who were overweight, hirsute, and relatively infertile with irregular or absent periods. Our knowledge of both the syndrome and its possible causes has increased as our ability to scan the ovary safely inside the pelvis and measure the level of various hormones has increased; but practice has not always entirely caught up with knowledge. The prevalence of polycystic ovaries in women without epilepsy has been described as being between 4–19% of potentially fertile women. It is important to remember that not all women with the syndrome are hairy, overweight, and with irregular menstruation; some women with the full syndrome are of normal weight and apparently normal menstruation but have disordered hormones.

The importance of the full syndrome is not just the effect it can have on fertility, important as that is, but also that women with it are particularly likely to develop type 2 diabetes in later life (and possibly be more prone to ovarian cancer).

## Why might women taking valproate sometimes have PCOS?

It may be connected to the fact that sodium valproate is known to have an effect on the metabolism of the pancreatic hormone insulin (lack of which causes diabetes). Insulin is involved in mediating ovarian function and in the causation of PCOS. Further Birmingham experience suggested that switching women with PCOS to another effective anticonvulsant and withdrawing the valproate led to the signs and symptoms of the PCOS disappearing and ovarian function returning to normal; the anticonvulsants used were levetiracetam and lamotrigine.

# Does the menstrual cycle affect epilepsy or its frequency?

Sometimes, but the answer is not completely straightforward. Some simple generalized absence epilepsies may disappear in female children at about the time that menstruation starts; but this may be no more than co-incidence as similar epilepsies stop in male children at about the same time.

However, some epilepsies probably do start at the same time as menstruation and become associated with the menstrual cycle, and may stop, or greatly diminish in frequency, during pregnancy and after the menopause. There is no doubt that in some women with epilepsy there is a close and tight relationship between the frequency of seizures and particular phases in the cycle. The problem is that the views of women with epilepsy and the views of physicians as to how commonly this association occurs vary greatly.

According to two recent studies, what can be said with some confidence is that between 10–12% of women with epilepsy have seizures in which all, or the vast majority, occur at a definite time in a regularly occurring menstrual cycle. This is almost always toward the latter end of the cycle just before or at the start of menstruation although there is a small number of a woman whose peak seizure frequency occurs at, or just before, ovulation in the middle of the cycle.

## What can be done about it?

It is usual to record seizure frequency and the menstrual cycle over 2 or 3 cycles—more if they are irregular. If it is then clear that a woman's seizures are related to her menstrual cycle:

◆ Sometimes regular anticonvulsant medication is enough; or taking clobazam or acetazolamide for up to a week at a defined point in the menstrual cycle can help.

◆ Hormone treatment like 'the pill' or the progesterone injection may be helpful (providing eventual pregnancy is not an issue), although rarely 'the pill' can worsen seizure frequency (see Chapter 11).

- Temporarily increasing the amount of anticonvulsant normally taken may rarely help, as can taking oral progesterone in the latter half of the menstrual cycle.

- Clomiphene has been suggested as a treatment for premenstrual seizures; this should only be used by experts as it can sometimes cause seizures.

- Switching off the menstrual cycle, with drugs such as goserelin, has also been recommended and does work, but can only ever be a temporary solution, as it is not usually prescribed for more than 6 months at a time.

The treatment of premenstrual seizures should be discussed with a medical advisor, as different patients will need different solutions (and the same patient may need different solutions at different times in her life).

#  Case study

**Sylvia** had her first tonic clonic seizure shortly after waking on the day of a maths exam at school ('I was never very good at it' she explained). She was swiftly investigated, given valproate, told she had juvenile myoclonic epilepsy, and that she would have to take anticonvulsants for the rest of her life.

She married at 25, continued to take 'the pill' until she was 28 and then stopped it to have a family. Some months after stopping 'the pill' her periods became very irregular and she often only had two or three a year but was told that was 'just her cycle'. After 11 years, at the age of 39 she still had not conceived (although her irregular cycle had raised the hope of pregnancy several times). She eventually requested specialist referral to an infertility clinic that had a contiguous epilepsy clinic.

Her EEG contained some generalized spike wave activity, particularly on overbreathing. MRI of her brain was normal, but MRI of her pelvis was not demonstrating severe polycystic ovaries: raised hormone levels demonstrated that she had PCOS. She was advised to switch to lamotrigine, which she did far more rapidly than the clinic intended—'time isn't on my side', she explained.

After being on lamotrigine for 6 months her periods became regular and her hormone levels had returned to normal. She was taking 5 milligrams of folic acid and conceived naturally and was seen in a joint obstetric/epilepsy clinic with regular blood level and EEG monitoring. At 38 weeks she chose to have an elective Caesarean section and had a healthy boy. She became pregnant again a year later delivering another healthy boy. She continues to take folic acid, chose not to breastfeed, sharing bottle feeding with her partner and at 44 is contemplating another pregnancy; 'I might have a girl, next time' she says, with a gleam in her eye—'I have a lot of catching up to do'. She has been advised to stop taking folic acid when she has decided that she has had enough children.

**10**

# Epilepsy and sexuality

 **Key points**

- Epilepsy should not interfere with the sexual life of women.
- Epilepsy related sexual feelings only seem to occur in women.
- Orgasm related seizures are rare—though many women fear them.
- If your seizures are induced by sexual activity you will usually have spontaneous ones as well.

Only rarely should epilepsy interfere with the sexual life of women. The sexual problems of women with epilepsy are, by and large, no different from those of women who do not have epilepsy except for the fear that if they 'let go', they will suffer a seizure. As a result their sexual response may become inhibited. This can usually be overcome by education and reassurance, which the sexual partner will often need as well.

The evidence about whether medication plays any part in dampening down sexual interest and arousal in women with epilepsy is sparse and contradictory but the consensus view is that it does not. The centres in the brain that are concerned with sexual interest and arousal are different between women and men, so that one cannot extrapolate data from one sex to the other.

 **Fact**

Although many women with epilepsy unnecessarily fear orgasm-related seizures, they are excessively rare.

One patient with orgasm-related, complex partial or tonic clonic seizures known to Tim claimed that sexual partners did not always notice that they had occurred—or perhaps were too polite or too embarrassed to say anything.

Epilepsy-related sexual feelings (a sexual feeling occurring as part of an epileptic attack, either as an 'aura' before a major seizure or as part of a simple or complex partial seizure) seem only to occur in women (probably because of the different brain centres involved). They are of sexual feelings or actual arousal, either a general feeling or sensations localized to the vaginal area (and then sometimes bizarrely just on one side).

It may, of course, take the patient some time to admit that such feelings occur; one of Tim's patients was only 7 years old when her complex partial seizures, accompanied by an initial warm vaginal sexual feeling, started. Initially she did not have the words to describe the experience. Later, she was too embarrassed to do so until, as she said, 'I knew you well enough to know that you wouldn't laugh when I told you. I sort of miss them now they are gone; they were rather exciting and warm even if the rest of the seizure wasn't.' She was later to say, however, as her life and experiences developed, 'but they weren't as good as the real thing'.

Most women who have seizures initiated by sexual activity usually have spontaneous seizures as well. Most (but not all) have seizure-related sexual feelings initiated by sexual activity or by the hyperventilation that often accompanies sexual arousal and excitement. It is important to note that the not uncommon undressing behaviour that may be part of a complex partial seizure is not sexually based. Non-epileptic seizures may also accompany sexual activity (they are, after all, often associated with a history of previous sexual abuse) and may need to be carefully distinguished from actual epilepsy.

So, if you have epilepsy and have perceived sexual problems or difficulties that you want to change, go to your GP and ask for a referral. Your treatment and prospects of a 'cure' should be no different from those of women without epilepsy. Be open with your therapist—take this book along if you need to—and remember that most sex therapy involves a couple rather than an individual, although there are exceptions.

If you are one of that very select group of women in whom sexual activity seems to trigger a seizure or seems to be part of the seizure itself, then don't be afraid to say so; those that Tim has encountered during his clinical practice almost always responded to the appropriate medical or surgical treatment, leaving the woman to enjoy her sexual self unencumbered. Some clinicians, indeed, believe that a full, active, and happy sexual life is, in itself, a pretty powerful anticonvulsant.

# 11

# Contraception, epilepsy, and epilepsy treatment

> ## ➔ Key points
>
> - Contraception is still (largely) a woman's issue.
> - Choice of contraceptive method should be reliable and suit you, but some methods are not advisable if you have epilepsy (e.g. 'safe period').
> - There are four questions for you (and your advisor) to consider (see below).
> - If you have epilepsy, every pregnancy should (as far as possible) be planned.

## Four important questions

Contraception is still largely a woman's issue, partly because most methods are woman orientated and partly because the consequences of failed contraception are more immediate and serious if one is a woman.

Effective contraception is particularly important if you have epilepsy because every pregnancy should be a planned one (see Chapter 13). The woman (preferably with her partner if she has one) should choose a method of contraception that best suits her mood, situation, and inclinations. However, there are some facts mainly related to the anticonvulsant medication she is taking that she must bear in mind; likewise epilepsy can have effects on the menstrual cycle (see Chapter 9) making some forms of contraception, such as relying on the 'safe period,' inadvisable. With the assistance of her professional advisor, she should try to answer the following questions.

- Will my epilepsy affect my use of this particular method of contraception?
- Will my epilepsy medication affect my method of contraception?
- Will my method of contraception affect my epilepsy?
- Will my method of contraception affect my anticonvulsant medication?

We will try to answer these questions, but do remember that ideas and information change so it is important that you also discuss these matters with a relevant health professional.

## Can epilepsy affect the use of any particular method of contraception?

Possibly, particularly if you have fairly frequent seizures, which may make your memory unreliable causing you, sometimes, to forget to take 'the pill'. Having a reliable partner, who can check for you and remind you, can help. However, if this does apply to you, perhaps consider a method of contraception like the Mirena coil or depot progestogen injections, which don't rely so heavily on your memory for their efficacy.

## Will my epilepsy medication affect my contraception?

Under certain circumstances, it can. The combined oral contraceptive's efficacy, which is very high when taken properly, is reduced by anticonvulsant medication which is 'enzyme inducing'. This means that the drug increases the amount of enzymes in the liver that break down other drugs, including oestrogen in the 'combined pill' thus lowering its efficiency.

When the dose of oestrogen in 'the pill' was reduced to 50 micrograms breakthrough bleeding (menstruating whilst still taking the active pill) began to occur in some women taking enzyme-inducing anticonvulsants as well (suggesting relative oestrogen component failure) and untoward pregnancies began to occur, particularly when the dose of oestrogen in the pill was reduced further (to 30 or 20 micrograms).

### The 'pill' and anticonvulsants

Knowledge of the interaction between certain anticonvulsants and the oestrogen in the pill was fairly slow to percolate through the medical profession. In an American study published just over 14 years ago, less than half of the neurologists and obstetricians polled knew of the effect that enzyme-inducing anticonvulsants might have on the pill. Only 4% of the neurologists could correctly identify which anticonvulsants were enzyme inducing and which were not (none of the obstetricians could). Over 20% of both reported contraceptive failures in their patients with epilepsy.

The enzyme-inducing anticonvulsant drugs are carbamazepine, oxcarbazepine, phenobarbital, phenytoin, primidone, topiramate, and zonisamide. (See Appendix 1 for detailed individual descriptions as intensity of induction varies.)

### What to do

If you are taking an enzyme-inducing anticonvulsant but wish to take an oral contraceptive, do not rely on it until you have slowly increased the dose of oestrogen in the pill over several months and until bleeding only occurs in the pill-free week.

This may be difficult with the modern low-dose oral contraceptives; even if a regular cycle is obtained the efficacy of the pill may not be complete (probably only 93% if you are taking carbamazepine for instance). This is still higher than a barrier method of contraception on its own, but if you want to be as sure that your contraception is reliable use a barrier method as well. The alternative solution would be to switch to an anticonvulsant drug that is not enzyme inducing but this may not be possible.

### Progestogen-only pills and injections

With the exception of phenobarbital, anticonvulsants should not cause problems with these. However, oral progesterone-only contraceptives have to be taken absolutely regularly to be effective (and even then are not quite as effective as the combined pill). Again, use with a barrier method for complete contraceptive confidence. Most authorities feel that blood levels of the progestogen injection are not affected by enzyme-inducing anticonvulsants, although to be on the safe side some, but not all, authorities suggest an injection every 10 rather than every 12 weeks.

## Will my method of contraception affect my epilepsy?

Oral contraceptives and injections may stop seizures, as various hormonal methods of contraception can be anticonvulsant in their own right, particularly in women with premenstrual seizures. The contraceptive is started and the seizures stop, only to return when it is withdrawn some years later, either when the relationship is over or the woman wants to start a family. The answer is to try to control the seizures before the contraceptive is started but this is not always possible and one does not want to deny the woman the most effective method of contraception, paradoxically particularly if she is still having seizures.

Occasionally, the opposite is true and the use of the contraceptive can be associated with an increase in seizure frequency. Sometimes this may be no more than a coincidence or related to anxiety caused by a change in life circumstances, but it may sometimes be caused by a depot injection of progesterone.

Emergency use of the 'morning-after pill' is safe if one has epilepsy, although if the person is taking enzyme-inducing medication a higher dose than usual may be needed.

## Contraception methods best avoided if you have epilepsy

◆ Sub-dermal (under the skin) hormonal implants—there is a potentially high failure rate for those with epilepsy.

◆ The Persona® and rhythm methods of contraception—since epilepsy can interfere with hormone cycles, and thus the timing of ovulation, such methods become even more unreliable than usual.

◆ The 'withdrawal method' of contraception, when the penis is suddenly yanked out of the vagina just before ejaculation—although it is without risk to epilepsy, it is a great risk to pregnancy.

### Condoms

The male method of contraception, the sheath, can be a reasonably effective method, particularly if combined with a spermicidal jelly or cream, providing that the user is practised in its use and only ever allows penetration when the protective is firmly in place.

### The IUD

The intrauterine device or 'coil' is an acceptable method of contraception if fitted properly particularly if it contains a locally-acting hormone (progesterone) as well, such as the Mirena coil. In women prone to seizures stretching the neck of the womb to insert the device may rarely cause a seizure, so the person inserting the coil should be aware of this possibility and have the necessary first aid to hand. It is usually only advised if you have already had a child.

### Will my method of contraception affect my anticonvulsant medication?

There is at least one example of a method of contraception affecting an anticonvulsant. Although lamotrigine does not affect the contraceptive pill, the combined pill can affect the blood level of lamotrigine (and possibly also valproate). If you are already taking lamotrigine in monotherapy and start taking the combined pill you should consider increasing your dose of lamotrigine by one-third to one-half, particularly if the dose you are taking is quite low. As always, it is something to be discussed with your medical advisor.

# 📄 Case study

**Zenobia** was 16 and had just started her 'A levels' when she began to experience episodes of briefly feeling frightened and detached from her surroundings; her best friend told her that for 2 or 3 minutes she would look 'strange' and would not answer if spoken to but merely mutter incomprehensibly. These episodes became frequent, but seemed only to occur in English lessons. The GP, puzzled by this, referred her to a nearby specialist unit where all examinations were found to be normal.

She had some English lessons with 24-hour EEG and ECG recorders in place. She had one of her attacks in a rather dry discourse on *Pride and Prejudice* closely followed by two others. The result was clear-cut spike wave EEG activity in her left temporal lobe. On 75 milligrams a day of lamotrigine the attacks stopped and she rapidly caught up in her studies, got a very good degree and came back to a local university to do research (in English).

Suddenly, after 4 seizure-free years she began to have repeats of her previous attacks. Once again all physical investigations were quite normal. A clue to the possible cause of the return of her seizures was found in the blood level of lamotrigine that had dropped to half of what it had been. Two months before, she had started to take the combined oral contraceptive pill. The dose was increased to 150 milligrams daily and the seizures stopped.

And the 'English lesson-induced' epilepsy? 'Actually,' she said, 'I had seizures in other places as well, but no one noticed and I wasn't going to say as they were really frightening; but your matter of fact approach to them made me lose my fear of them.'

# 12

# Epilepsy and fertility

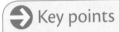 Key points

- Infertility (not having a pregnancy after 2 years of regular trying) is common.
- Some women with epilepsy may be less fertile than the average woman.
- Women with epilepsy have more anovulatory (eggless) menstrual cycles.
- Get your epilepsy and child-friendly medication sorted BEFORE infertility treatment.
- Premature menopause is possibly commoner in women with epilepsy.

## Definition and frequency

- *Relative infertility*—a couple having regular intercourse are not thought to be infertile until they have been trying unsuccessfully for 2 years.
- *Absolute infertility*—never becoming pregnant, at least without medical assistance.

Both types of infertility are surprisingly common, affecting at least one in six couples in the UK, and is said to be increasing with male sperm counts slowly falling. This may be because women are on average delaying their first pregnancy until much later in life. Whatever the reason, fertility in women with epilepsy is said to be less than that of women who do not have epilepsy. There may be several reasons for this, depending on the population studied.

Some women with epilepsy have other handicaps that make pregnancy difficult if not impossible. But in an extensive population study the evidence seemed clear enough that the fertility rate of women with epilepsy, when other factors were taken into account, was less than that of women who did not have epilepsy. Women with epilepsy, particularly if still having seizures, are more prone to anovulatory menstrual cycles as already mentioned, polycystic ovaries, and PCOS.

It is possible that some women with epilepsy deliberately choose to remain childless but nowadays we would hold that to be unnecessary unless the woman is suffering from a known rare genetic disorder particularly if she has undergone pre-conception counselling when such issues and risks will have been explored.

## Get the epilepsy sorted first

It seems nonsensical that expensive and stressful infertility treatment is carried out before questions about the epilepsy, its investigation, its most advantageous treatment, and the use of folic acid have been settled and acted upon, which may take some time. Yet in a group of women with epilepsy referred to a local infertility clinic (and therefore referred on to our contiguous women's epilepsy service) this had never been done and some referrers expressed surprise that it should be thought necessary. Yet, in this small group, one woman turned out not to have epilepsy at all and three (see the Case study of Sylvia in Chapter 9) originally taking valproate began to menstruate normally when switched to a different anticonvulsant and became pregnant naturally. The type of intervention that the fertility clinic proposes needs to be discussed with the epilepsy service in case there is a possible interaction between gynaecological and epileptic therapies.

## Premature menopause

Premature menopause, the end of the periods occurring before the age of 40, may be commoner in women with epilepsy. One American study has suggested it with fairly compelling evidence but we need a more detailed large number study with appropriate controls to be sure. The experience of the Birmingham clinic was that there may be some truth in the finding and we suggested as a prudent rule that women with epilepsy should try to have their first child by the time they reached the age of 30.

# 13

# Preconception counselling for women with epilepsy

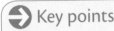 Key points

Before trying to become pregnant, consult your medical advisor and work out:

- Whether your epilepsy has been fully and appropriately investigated.
- The medication best suited to the baby and to the control of your seizures.
- Any perceived difficulties you may have in becoming pregnant (e.g. irregular periods).
- If surgery is a possibility then it is best done before pregnancy starts.

Before becoming pregnant (at least a couple of years before if drug changes are contemplated) a woman with epilepsy needs to sit down with her medical advisor to decide her optimum plan for her epilepsy and the forthcoming pregnancy in terms of both the medication she will need and any untoward effect it may have on the pregnancy and any perceived difficulties she may have in becoming pregnant. What she decides to do will to a large extent depend on the control she already has over her seizures and the medication she is currently taking.

## Is this really epilepsy?

Diagnosis is not always easy and opinions may change. There have been several recent accounts of women who did not have epilepsy being treated as though they did and having anticonvulsant damaged babies as a result so it is worthwhile reviewing. How was the diagnosis arrived at and has anything happened since to possibly alter it? What investigations were done and are more needed? Usually, of course, the decision that it is clearly epilepsy will be unaltered.

# Is it safe to withdraw from medication?

If possible, this would be best for the unborn child. The chances of successful withdrawal depend on the type of epilepsy and how long a woman has been seizure free. A fairly recent British study tried to look at this question by taking a group of people whose epilepsy had rapidly come under control with the first anticonvulsant tried, who had then remained seizure free for some years, and who did not have an obvious structural cause in their brains to account for the epilepsy. Half were slowly withdrawn from their anticonvulsant drug; the other half stayed on medication. At the end of the study 20% of those who withdrew from medication began to have seizures again. This may seem a high number but almost the same number of the 'continued treatment' group also relapsed during the trial. Looked at another way, the majority of people with epilepsy who rapidly become seizure free and remain so and who do not have a cerebral lesion can safely withdraw from medication; most of those patients who did have fresh seizures gained control again easily when medication was restarted.

Those people who have had successful surgery for their epilepsy can also usually withdraw slowly from medication after a year or so. Do bear in mind that your specialists may well have different ideas and new evidence may present itself after this book is written, so discuss with them what is best for you and your individual case.

# If seizures start again can they be controlled again?

Generally, yes. However, seizures can sometimes be more difficult to control second time around. If seizures do recur, it is a good idea to fully investigate the epilepsy again in case a physical cause is now more obvious. It is also a good idea to get them under control as quickly as possible again, using a drug like levetiracetam in which a therapeutic dose can be used from the start (other drugs like valproate and phenytoin which can be used in this way are not advisable in those trying to become pregnant). Sadly, delay in treating seizures that have recurred in patients seizure free and taken off medication has been fatal due to SUDEP.

# How to withdraw?

- If you are going to withdraw from medication (and never do this without discussing the pros and cons with your medical advisor) it must be done slowly over several months.

- If you are taking more than one drug then withdraw from one drug completely before tackling the next one.

- The withdrawal period will be slower and longer if the drug is being taken in monotherapy.

- With some drugs (like valproate) seizures may possibly not return for some months after withdrawal.

◆ If you have an epilepsy which has been difficult to control or which has a known cause (like hippocampal sclerosis—see Chapter 1) then withdrawal is much more problematic, even if you are only on one drug and your seizures are well controlled.

◆ It may be better sometimes to switch to a more pregnancy-friendly drug than withdrawing altogether.

# Has my epilepsy been fully investigated?

This depends on the type of epilepsy the person has. If there is clear evidence that it was simple absence epilepsy, then the only investigation needed would be an EEG with appropriate overbreathing; but, in that case, the seizures should have long since stopped and the medication been withdrawn before the question of pregnancy comes up. If it is not simple benign epilepsy, has sufficient EEG and good quality MRI investigation been done to establish its type and cause? If yes, are you confident the details have been explained to you and you are fully in the picture (if not, make sure someone does explain them to you)? If your epilepsy has not been fully diagnosed and investigated before you get pregnant, even if you are seizure free, this should be done before you try to become pregnant.

 Case study

**Andrea** had been seizure free for a couple of years and became pregnant after having one (normal) EEG; 5 months into the pregnancy she began to have complex partial seizures again and an MRI (which was said to have been 'unnecessary' in the face of a normal EEG—that is not true) revealed a benign tumour that was slowly expanding because of the pregnancy. Luckily it was possible to remove it surgically after she had delivered and the pregnancy survived, but the tumour should have been recognized and the surgery carried out before she got pregnant.

It is important to recognize and deal with lesions before pregnancy, particularly because successful surgery may mean that anticonvulsants can eventually be withdrawn and previously unrecognized vascular lesions (see Chapter 2) can rupture or bleed for the first time during pregnancy with disastrous results.

# Staying on medication—what next?

If your medical advisor decides that the risk of withdrawing from medication is too high, it is usually still possible to reduce the burden of anticonvulsant drug the woman is taking. This can reduce the risk of the medication doing harm to the pregnancy. One study found that it was often possible to reduce the dosage of anticonvulsant by reducing the number of drugs the woman is on (if she is taking more than one). This has to be done slowly and one tries to withdraw the drug most likely to cause birth defects (thus sodium valproate is withdrawn whilst carbamazepine remains). The blood level of some drugs may alter if the other is removed and may need to be adjusted during the withdrawal process. But, if you possibly can, take just one anticonvulsant drug before trying to become pregnant. Remember, the dose may have to go up whilst you are pregnant (see Chapter 14).

## I am still having seizures, what should I do?

Discuss with your medical advisor whether, with a change of medication, you could become seizure free before becoming pregnant. A recent British survey suggested that this might often be possible. If you cannot become seizure free it is best to enter pregnancy taking as little medication as possible, consistent with safety, and avoiding certain anticonvulsants if possible (see Appendix 1). Although a mother's tonic clonic seizures have been reported to have a transient effect on the heart rate of the baby in the womb, and briefly on its metabolism, there is no direct evidence that they seriously damage the baby's health (although seizures late in pregnancy may have an effect on the mother's well being due to the greater likelihood of inhalation of vomit into the lungs). Partial seizures are reported to have no effect.

## Avoid status epilepticus

Status epilepticus is particularly dangerous, both for mother and child, and should be avoided as much as possible and treated rapidly if it does occur. Women with epilepsy should ideally be delivered in hospital (a point we will discuss again in Chapter 15) and be looked after during the pregnancy by a combined epilepsy and obstetric team wherever possible, and where not possible by teams that have a close communication and dialogue. Remember also to take 5 milligrams of folic acid by mouth daily, if you can for at least a year before becoming pregnant (see Chapter 7).

## What about the rest of your health?

A preconception health check means looking at other aspects of your life and health as well and making any changes that may be necessary; this means alcohol, general health, and weight (being markedly overweight or underweight can impair your fertility).

It is better to stop drinking before you try to become pregnant as alcohol damage to the baby occurs early, before you may realise that you are pregnant. There is clear guidance from the UK government that alcohol should be avoided in pregnancy, which is probably right as you are already taking medication that may have its own effect on the baby (see Appendix 1).

# 14

# Epilepsy and pregnancy

 Key points

- If you fall pregnant unexpectedly DON'T stop or reduce your anticonvulsants.

- Tablet taking needs to work round early nausea and vomiting.

- Make sure you have all the appropriate tests and scans of the baby.

- If you have an unexpected seizure in pregnancy be certain that it is not 'eclampsia'.

- Early miscarriage is common but no more so in women with epilepsy.

- Late miscarriage needs investigating and possible preventative treatment.

- At about 32 weeks decision needs to be made about method of delivery. Women with 'brittle' epilepsy may need an elective Caesarean section.

- Co-operation between GP, epilepsy specialist, and obstetrician is vital.

## Don't worry if you've been caught out

We were saying in the last chapter that it is better, if you have epilepsy, that you have planned and thought about your pregnancy, but human nature being what it is you may, of course, be pregnant unexpectedly. It is sad, but true, that if any damage to your baby has been caused as a result of the medication you are taking, which is by no means certain, it has probably already happened by the time you realise that you are pregnant. Seek specialist advice straight away and work out what is the best thing to do in your particular situation, making sure that you have the necessary scans and assessments.

> If you are pregnant and are reading this chapter with a mounting feeling of dread don't despair! Whatever else you do, do NOT suddenly stop your anticonvulsant medication, as that is very dangerous.
>
> Sudden death in epilepsy is, unfortunately, a risk in pregnancy and we suspect that one of the main causes is an unprepared woman with epilepsy stopping her medication abruptly.

The risk to your child, even if you are not taking folic acid at conception and are on medication is not all that high. If severe damage is present (like spina bifida) it can be detected at a stage in the pregnancy where you can decide whether to terminate it or not.

If you are still having seizures it would be worthwhile trying to control them during the pregnancy if possible, so discuss that with your epilepsy specialist. Choose, if possible, medication that is 'safe' for the baby and which can be given in a therapeutic dose from the start like levetiracetam. If there is a good reason for it, a head MRI can also be obtained whilst you are pregnant, as can EEGs.

## Does epilepsy sometimes start in pregnancy?

Yes, it can, although sometimes the epilepsy has started before the pregnancy but has gone unrecognized. Since epilepsy can start at any age it is not unreasonable that it will sometimes start when a woman is pregnant. The commonest time for pregnancy-related epilepsy to start is shortly after the birth when fatigue is added to metabolic changes. If epilepsy starts in pregnancy or shortly afterwards it needs immediate investigation (since blood vessel abnormalities may present with epilepsy for the first time in pregnancy) and rapid treatment to get it under control as quickly as possible with support in place during the exhausting adjustment that every woman goes through with the advent of a new child, and now with the added burden of the newly arrived epilepsy (see Chapter 16).

## A seizure during pregnancy—is it eclampsia?

There is an added complication to epilepsy (particularly if tonic clonic) occurring in pregnancy, particularly in the later stages, called eclampsia. Let's explain. During pregnancy your blood pressure will be measured on many occasions and your ankles checked for swelling; a rise in blood pressure (beyond strictly defined limits) or sudden ankle swelling is a sign of pre-eclampsia. If the blood pressure continues to rise and the other metabolic causes of the condition continue unchecked, eclampsia (tonic clonic seizures—eclamptic fits) will supervene. These are dangerous to both mother and child and have to be brought under control quickly. If these warning signs occur you will be encouraged to rest in bed (which usually means that the signs settle down again) but if blood pressure rises higher then it will be suggested that the baby is delivered early since this is safer for you and the baby.

Obstetricians take the prevention of eclampsia very seriously. A tonic clonic seizure occurring after the 20th week of pregnancy without a concomitant rise in blood pressure or ankle swelling, in someone with a known history of epilepsy, is very unlikely to be eclampsia. However, the obstetric team (not to mention you) will need a lot of reassurance that it is not.

There is absolutely no evidence to suggest that pre-eclampsia or eclampsia is more common in women with epilepsy than in the general population of women; if you have had pre-eclampsia in one pregnancy there is a risk that it may return in the next and subsequent pregnancies although it is more likely that it will not. If you have epilepsy, or a history of it, it is clearly important to monitor blood pressure closely and to deal with pre-eclampsia and threatened eclampsia energetically.

## But, OK, I'm pregnant—now what?

◆ See your doctor straightaway and have the pregnancy confirmed and referral to an obstetric hospital with the necessary expertise and links to your epilepsy specialist (this may not be the nearest one to you geographically).

◆ You may not actually attend the clinic until you are 10–12 weeks pregnant unless there is some other problem that needs assessing early (one woman seen by Tim had insulin-dependent diabetes and an active collagen disorder (inflammation of the body's connective tissue) in addition to epilepsy—she had much monitoring but eventually a normal baby).

◆ Sometimes, you may be seen early if there is doubt about your expected date of delivery or your epilepsy is particularly severe.

◆ At the first visit a general medical history and examination will be done, plus a gynaecological and, if relevant, obstetric history. This is when your epilepsy will be discussed and arrangements should be made for it to be monitored during the pregnancy, whether you are having seizures or not, or taking medication or not.

◆ The number of times you will be seen in the specialist clinic whilst you are pregnant will depend upon your epilepsy and your obstetric needs.

## Miscarriage

Some pregnancies do, sadly, end in a miscarriage. Neither early nor late miscarriage is any commoner in women with epilepsy than would be expected by chance. Most are early on in the pregnancy (indeed the woman may not even realise she is pregnant but just assumes that her period is a little later and heavier than normal).

- *Early miscarriage* is fairly common and, although unfortunate for the woman involved, does not mean there is anything wrong with her. She will be encouraged to 'try again' in due course.

- *Recurrent early miscarriage* can be due to an unsuspected illness in the mother that needs investigating and can often be corrected; epilepsy itself is not one of these diseases but rarely the underlying cause of the epilepsy can be.

- *Miscarriage after the 12th week* of pregnancy, when the placenta forms and embeds itself in the lining of the womb is much less common and is sometimes due, particularly if recurrent, to a defect in the neck of the womb that prevents it from closing properly so that the developing fetus falls out (the so-called 'incompetent cervix'); this can be corrected by stitching the neck of the womb which then has to be undone when the woman goes into labour.

## Scans and other investigations

*At about the 12th week* of pregnancy an ultrasound scan of the womb is done; this is the dating scan that accurately foretells the age of the pregnancy (and sometimes reveals there is more than one occupant of the womb).

*At about the 18th week* another scan is done to evaluate the structure of the fetus at a time when, if there is something wrong like spina bifida, the parents can decide whether to continue with the pregnancy or not. This scan is important if you have epilepsy so make sure it is done.

*Blood tests*—you will have had routine blood tests, looking particularly for anaemia, which is common in pregnancy and may need to be corrected. You may be offered a blood test for hepatitis and AIDS depending on your previous history and lifestyle (don't be offended; specialists are thinking about both your health and that of your baby). Your blood group will be determined and whether you are Rhesus positive or negative (which may have an effect on the baby's health in the womb but can be dealt with). If appropriate, blood levels of your anticonvulsants will also be measured (see later) and a plan of future antenatal visits and tests worked out.

A blood test is now routinely done to estimate the risk of Down syndrome; it is also possible to do a 'nuchal scan' (of the neck of the fetus in the womb) at about 14 weeks to detect a reliable sign of the child having Down syndrome. This is a new and accurate test. If the risk is felt to be high, at about 18 weeks of pregnancy an amniocentesis can be carried out (taking a small amount of the fluid that surrounds the developing fetus in the womb and analysing it). However, this carries a small but definite risk of producing a late miscarriage, so it should only be done after a full discussion of the potential risks and benefits with your consultant. Once again there is no evidence that epilepsy itself has any influence on whether or not a child has Down syndrome.

# What sort of delivery?

*At 32 weeks* of pregnancy it is usual to have a consultation about the best way of ensuring a healthy delivery of the child. You and your doctor could decide to:

- Allow nature to take her course.
- Aim for a spontaneous natural vaginal delivery.
- Induce labour and speed up and assist delivery.
- Choose a Caesarean section, either when labour starts or at a defined point in the pregnancy.

Nature, of course, has a habit of altering these plans unexpectedly but there is evidence that for women with epilepsy a labour lasting no more than about 12 hours is best to avoid exhaustion and an increased risk of seizures. Sometimes a planned Caesarean section may be best. We will discuss delivery itself and the important topic of pain relief in Chapter 15.

# Will my seizures return or get worse?

This is not an easy question to answer because it depends on the person. The usually quoted old statistic is that in a third of women there will be no change in seizure frequency, in a third it will be less, and in a third more than usual. This much quoted figure conceals more than it explains—and what of the woman who enters pregnancy seizure free; can she remain so?

There are two things that are fairly certain:

- Women who have genuine pre-menstrual epilepsy will tend to lose their seizures whilst they are pregnant; this is not invariable but likely enough.
- Seizures are more likely to occur in pregnancy in women with epilepsy whose pre-pregnancy anticonvulsant blood levels were low.

Additionally, it is likely that women who attend a specialist clinic regularly whilst pregnant and in whom swift changes can be made in dose and type of medication if necessary are more likely to remain seizure free; but this is still supposition and has not been 'proved' in a properly conducted trial.

# What bodily changes does pregnancy cause?

Pregnancy exerts marked changes in the body and the way it functions that may have an effect on epilepsy and its drug treatment, sometimes unpredictably. Women with epilepsy unprepared for pregnancy may deliberately stop their medication, which, as indicated previously, is very dangerous, and may lead to status epilepticus with consequent loss of the child. In Tim's experience women who have done this have not totally stopped their medication but have withdrawn from some of it; this is equally dangerous and cannot be advised. For some medications like valproate, maintaining the same dose but spreading it over 4 times a day is sometimes suggested to avoid peak blood levels.

## Nausea and vomiting—pregnancy sickness

This often blights the first few months of pregnancy. It is often called morning sickness although can sometimes be at its peak at other times of the day or night.

◆ If you are sick within an hour of taking your anticonvulsant medication (particularly if you recognize your tablets or fragments of them in what you bring up) then take the dose again.

◆ Since the vomiting (if not the nausea) tends to peak at certain definite times of the day it is usually possible to adjust the time you take your tablets to a safer time of the day; discuss this with your medical advisor if necessary.

◆ It is better, since you are taking medication already, not to take other drugs to control the vomiting of pregnancy but, if you develop the severe and excessive vomiting of pregnancy that sometimes occurs for not very obvious reasons, then this must be treated as a medical emergency and you may have to take anti sickness medication (usually by injection) whilst being admitted to hospital. The condition usually settles quickly with appropriate treatment.

## Drug absorption and metabolism

During pregnancy the stomach becomes more inert (in other words the constant muscular contractions and relaxations of the stomach wall diminish markedly) so that absorption of a drug through its walls may be less efficient. The volume of plasma in the blood stream increases by about 50% at its peak and the amount of blood pumped from the heart increases by about 30%, meaning it has to work much harder. The amount of water in the body tissues also increases (this means that a given dose of a drug may be less absorbed and, once absorbed, more diluted in the blood stream than normal). The way the liver works also changes; the proteins that bind foreign substances (including drugs) to themselves to inactivate them reduce in quantity, which means that more drug able to react may be present in the blood stream than usual. Add to this the common sleep deprivation that occurs in pregnancy and several reasons occur which may increase seizure frequency (and one or two that may decrease it) making prediction difficult as to what is likely to happen in response to a given dose of a drug.

## Drug blood levels—useful or not?

The literature on this subject is somewhat sparse, a little conflicting and largely confined to older drugs like phenobarbital and phenytoin. It is important to know what the blood level was before the pregnancy started, and that all levels before, during, and after the pregnancy are measured at the same time interval after the drug has been taken. Blood levels of both carbamazepine and lamotrigine consistently fall during pregnancy, usually stabilizing after week 32. It was Tim's policy to increase the dose of both drugs to keep the measured blood level the same as before the pregnancy started. This never gave rise to the easily recognized side effects of too much of either drug and did mean that patients treated in this way remained seizure free, with monthly measuring of blood levels and swift dose adjustments accordingly. It is important to note here that this is not a decision that every specialist would make, so you will have to ask your local team what policy they follow. It also means that drug doses had to be reduced, often quite rapidly, when the baby had been delivered. Ask your doctor what side effects to look out for.

But what of those drugs whose blood level is not usually measured? Should one increase the dose anyway, or wait until the patient, if seizure free, has a seizure? Fortunately for many people with epilepsy, even those long seizure free, there may be other indications that a seizure is near—'I feel fitty' as one patient phrased it. The return of early morning waking jerks, brief lapses of concentration, or other changes in an individual may warn that a seizure is near and medication therefore can be increased appropriately. One must be careful to distinguish these warning signs and symptoms from understandable feelings of anxiety and apprehension (unless they themselves are a known precursor of a seizure in a particular individual). This means that, if possible, the specialist must know the patient well and give her enough time and confidence to air these feelings and fears that are often difficult to articulate.

Finally, no matter how supportive her medical team, a woman with epilepsy may well be asking herself, until it is born and in her arms, 'is my baby really alright?' (regardless of how many times she has been told that it is!). This thought may never be articulated but may take many months to fully assuage. A woman with epilepsy whilst pregnant and after the birth needs a great deal of support. In the next chapter we will consider the birth itself and the potential consequences for it of having epilepsy.

##  Case study

**Janine** was 12 when she began to experience jerks of her legs within an hour of waking; at 14, during a period she had a tonic clonic seizure. She was taken to hospital, given valproate and told, after a normal EEG, that she had juvenile myoclonic epilepsy and would need to take valproate for a very long time (but was not told why). At 22 she married and, before trying for her first child sensibly requested advice about epilepsy, medication, and pregnancy. A nurse specialist told her (a) that valproate was as safe as any drug in pregnancy (not true) and (b) there was no convincing evidence that folic acid should be taken before trying to become pregnant (also not true).

Reassured, Janine returned home; her periods were very irregular but after 3 years she finally became pregnant. Sadly an 18-week ultrasound showed that the child had a severe spina bifida and she reluctantly accepted the offered termination.

She changed her GP and requested specialist referral elsewhere. Her epilepsy was reassessed and juvenile myoclonic epilepsy was confirmed (the nature of the syndrome and the need to remain on medication was carefully explained). She was accordingly slowly transferred to lamotrigine and the valproate withdrawn; on a dose of lamotrigine of 100 milligrams a day she remained seizure free and with a normal 24-hour EEG.

She lost 2 stone in weight and her periods became regular with normal hormone blood levels. She started to take 5 milligrams of folic acid every day and, with some trepidation, became pregnant 3 months later. She was seen monthly in a joint obstetric/epilepsy clinic and detailed scans of the child were reported as perfectly normal; lamotrigine doses were adjusted according to blood levels in the usual way and she had a normal delivery of a healthy boy at 38 weeks and had a normal delivery of a healthy girl 2 years later.

---

The pregnancies of all women with epilepsy in the United Kingdom, whatever the outcome, should be reported to:

The Epilepsy and Pregnancy Register
The Royal Hospitals
Grosvenor Road
Belfast
BT12 6BA
Free phone 0800 389 1248

Do encourage your doctor to help with this, as it is the only way we will truly know the answer to many of the questions posed in this book. If you are from elsewhere in Europe there is a Europe wide register (EURAP) contactable at the same address. Similar research is carried out elsewhere in the world (contact Epilepsy Action (appendix two) for details).

# 15

# Labour, birth, and the immediate aftermath in women with epilepsy

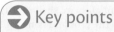 **Key points**

- Labour may be natural, induced, speeded up, or circumvented.
- Labour, and its immediate aftermath, is the most likely time to have a seizure but this can almost invariably be prevented with a little thought.
- Women with epilepsy often fear labour and 'losing control'.
- They shouldn't have the baby at home—despite its advantages.
- Take a copy of a summary of your epilepsy care with you (unless shared clinic).
- Take some of your epilepsy medication with you and make sure you get it on time
- Make sure the obstetric unit knows what to do if you have a seizure (there should be a plan).
- Make sure there is a plan in case of frequent vomiting in labour.

## So it's started—OK, but read this first!

It is best to have read this chapter, and discussed any issues that it raises with your medical advisor, before you go into labour. You should have made a plan at your clinic visit around the 32nd week of your pregnancy. The plan must take account of the fact that labour and its immediate aftermath is the most likely time to have a seizure if you have epilepsy. This increased risk of having seizures has several causes, most of which are preventable with a little thought but some of which are not.

The first thing to say is that women with epilepsy, even when it is well controlled, fear labour more than women who do not have epilepsy. Having discussed this with many women we think it may have a little to do with the increased risk of seizures but mainly probably to do with the fear of temporarily losing that tight control over oneself that many women with epilepsy adopt as a defence mechanism. Proper preparation allays much of this understandable fear but is something that professionals, who have 'seen it all before' must acknowledge. So, labour has started (or your waters have broken), and you are about to go to hospital; what is the plan?

## Why can't I have the baby at home?

In some ways home as a place to give birth may have advantages; less stress, less risk of infection, a familiar midwife, supportive relatives, a less medical atmosphere, and sometimes even a GP who is obstetrically trained. But home has a distinct disadvantage; lack of immediate access to an anaesthetist and a paediatrician to look after you if your epilepsy gets out of control. To give the best chance to your baby, hospital delivery, despite the drawbacks of birth among strangers, is best. Under certain circumstances it is essential, as we shall shortly see. So, if you are very keen on a home birth, do discuss the pros and cons with your medical advisor very carefully.

## What should you take with you?

One doesn't always wait until labour has started before going into hospital; nowadays labour may be induced or circumvented. Let's assume that you are going into your chosen maternity unit either for an elective induction of labour (or an elective Caesarean operation) or are already in labour; what should you take with you?

### A brief written outline of your epilepsy

This should be written with and endorsed by both your epilepsy and obstetric services with a copy already in your notes. It is best to have more than one copy because it is amazing how quickly even important documents get lost in a busy hospital. It should include:

- The kind of seizures you have.
- How often they are likely to occur.
- What to do if they do happen or become too frequent.
- The results of investigations and your current medication (with a note about any dose increases in this pregnancy and what you have been told about any necessary dose reduction after the birth).

### Enough of your usual medication to cover your time in hospital

This is against normal hospital practice but, particularly if you are taking one of the newer anticonvulsants like lamotrigine or levetiracetam, you cannot assume that the unit's pharmacy will stock it and it may be a little while before they can obtain it. You, or your partner, will also have to ensure that your medication is taken at the time it is supposed to be (or as close to it as possible) and regularly and not assume that the midwives, with other things on their mind, will remember. Things may well be different if you are in a pre-delivery bed (in what used to be called a 'lying in' ward) or if you have to spend a few days in hospital post-delivery. Don't assume either that the doctors you meet will know much about your anticonvulsant medication so do make sure that your epilepsy team knows that you are in hospital as soon as you or the obstetric team can. Include a note of this on your epilepsy fact sheet.

## Should I have a Caesarean section?

For some women with epilepsy, particularly those still having seizures or whose epilepsy is 'brittle', an elective Caesarean section operation is best; this is usually done at the 38th week of the pregnancy before labour starts. It is done under the best possible circumstances for both mother and child (and not done in the middle of the night after an exhausting labour has failed with the child in distress). However, Caesarean section, even when done electively, is not without drawbacks involving a longer recovery time, a longer stay in hospital, possibly increased difficulty in bonding to the baby after the birth, and a scar in the womb that slightly weakens its future integrity (so much so that most women are allowed only three such operations). There may also be obstetric reasons for an elective Caesarean operation but it certainly should not be seen as a panacea despite its endorsement by those 'too posh to push'.

## Should my labour be 'induced' (started artificially)?

An 'induction' of labour, usually by 'breaking the waters' (cutting a hole in the amniotic sac that surrounds the baby in the womb) is appropriate in some cases. Having done this, if labour fails to start or proceeds too slowly or ineffectually, either an assisted delivery with the forceps or the ventouse (a suction device fitted to the top of the baby's oncoming head and then carefully pulled) or an emergency Caesarean section will be necessary. Often a drip is put into your arm at the same time with a drug in it that will induce and/or strengthen contractions. Labour is often shortened but effective pain relief will be necessary and a careful eye kept on you.

> As a general rule if you have epilepsy labour should last no longer than about 12 hours to avoid exhaustion (which increases the chance of having a seizure).

There may be exceptions to this bold statement; if you are well on into the second stage of labour, for instance, when the 12 hours are up (in other words the cervix—the neck of the womb—is fully dilated and the baby progressing satisfactorily into the birth canal) then one can wait a little longer for nature to take her course. If the cervix is not yet fully dilated and labour is not progressing properly then some kind of operative interference may be needed in order that the labour comes to a successful conclusion. Your first labour is likely to be the longest. 'Induction' is something that you must discuss with your obstetric team.

## Vomiting during labour—what to do

Some women are prone to vomit during labour. This usually doesn't matter and does not presage anything serious but, as already discussed in Chapter 14, can be a problem if you have epilepsy and have just taken your tablets for the day. If vomiting occurs within about an hour of ingesting your dose, particularly if fragments of your medication can be seen, then take them again.

## Pain relief

- The key to pain relief is prior practice (e.g. gas and air).
- Even if encouraged to, **don't** pant or over breathe.
- Some authorities think pethidine (a pain killer) is best avoided (there are others that can be used).
- TENS (transcutaneous electrical neural stimulation) machines can be helpful but need prior practice.
- Epidurals are good and safe.
- Have an agreed plan (between the epilepsy and obstetric unit) about when to use clobazam.

Most women will be offered 'gas and air' during contractions. This involves inhaling, through a mask, a mixture of nitrous oxide (laughing gas) and air, which deadens the pain of the contraction. Used properly it can be very helpful, reducing pain to bearable proportions and even allowing a wan smile to break out. Unfortunately few women are taught, prior to labour, how to use it properly so they pant like a dog when the mask is on their face; as a result only a little of the gas gets into the lungs making it ineffective. The trick is to use the mask and breathe deeply and slowly just before the contraction starts which some women learn to time well. Gas and air is quite safe to use if you have epilepsy providing **you do not pant** (since that is over breathing which can, of course, make a seizure more likely); in the heat of the moment this can be difficult to remember unless you have had practice in this technique.

In the second stage of labour listen carefully to what the midwife is telling you, but be selective in your response. When she shouts 'push right down into your bottom' then push like hell: but if she forgets and shouts 'now pant like a little dog' when the contraction is over then politely ignore her; people prone to seizures should not over breathe.

### Other methods of pain relief

*TENS machines* are used successfully for chronic pain syndromes and there is a vogue for using them to dull or relieve the pains of labour. Again, they need practice and experience to be really effective, but are quite safe to use if you have epilepsy.

*Epidural anaesthesia* The most effective pain relief in labour is epidural anaesthesia (an injection of local anaesthetic just outside the spinal cord in the lower back). This usually takes away the pain altogether but needs someone very skilled to inject it properly and, since you have lost all sensation, competent midwives to accurately check the various stages of the labour. Since you have lost the pain stimulus to push, a 'lift out' with the forceps is often needed at the end to facilitate delivery and you will remain somewhat numb down below for sometime afterwards. The pain relief is, however, very effective and there is good audited evidence that, in skilled hands, the procedure is quite safe in women with epilepsy; this, as ever, is something to discuss with your obstetrician.

## Should I have a local or general anaesthetic?

*Local anaesthetic* If you have an 'operative delivery' (forceps or the ventouse) or you need a small cut in your perineum (bottom) to avoid a tear in this delicate if somewhat overstretched area as the baby's head comes through then it is usual to use local anaesthetic injections to deaden the pain.

*General anaesthetic* If you are being offered a Caesarean section it is better for you to have a general anaesthetic than lots of local anaesthetic with the potential risk of inducing a seizure if too much is used; discuss this with the anaesthetist. You will miss the thrilling experience of your newborn infant being handed across the screen to your waiting arms but it is probably better to play safe.

## Should I take additional medication in labour (i.e. clobazam)

Should you take additional medication for 2–3 days over labour and the birth to protect you against having seizures—in other words some doses of clobazam if you are likely to have seizures especially if tired or stressed (if your epilepsy is 'brittle' or not well controlled then we have already suggested an elective Caesarean operation)? Obstetricians were initially against it because, as they rightly pointed out, the child when born would be somewhat sleepy and, perhaps for a few hours unable to suckle. We agreed, but argued that a seizure during labour or delivery might also have implications for the child's health and also for the mother's and that it was probably best to prevent it if possible. After much discussion it was agreed that a few mothers might be encouraged to use, say, 10 milligrams of clobazam twice daily for no more than 2 or 3 days over the delivery period and often less than that, but only after careful thought and agreement. As it turned out this proved to be very rarely necessary and those few babies born to mothers who did use clobazam were not overly sleepy anyway.

## If a seizure occurs what is the best thing to do?

1–2% of women with epilepsy will have a seizure during delivery, although many can probably be prevented. The best course of action depends on what kind of seizure occurred and whether it is likely to be repeated:

*Simple or complex partial seizures* are unlikely to be repeated and little need be done since it will be very unlikely to have affected the baby or the course of the delivery. However, if the seizures look likely to be repeated or partial status develops then the uterus should be evacuated as quickly as possible (by emergency Caesarean operation, forceps, or ventouse extraction) and the mother given oral clobazam or intravenous diazepam.

*A tonic clonic seizure* occurring in labour means urgent consideration must be given to sedating the mother and evacuating her uterus as quickly as possible, particularly if the fetal heart rate falls (as it usually will, for about half an hour). Once the baby is safely delivered then a decision can be made about whether to continue sedation for a day or two. Again the obstetricians will need to be sure that the seizure was truly that of the woman's usual epilepsy and not related to eclampsia.

## After the birth

The mother is moved to the post-delivery ward and tries to sleep whilst the baby yells its head off and demands to be fed. There is evidence that the mother remains at an increased risk of seizures (again perhaps 1–2%) for another 48 hours or so. This risk can be much reduced by making sure that she gets her usual dose of anticonvulsant at the usual time (proud new father, are you awake?) and gets enough sleep. The obstetrician will be concerned at this time that a seizure could still be one of eclampsia.

If the woman has decided to breastfeed (see Table 15.1 and Appendix 1 for detailed information about which drugs are safe for breastfeeding and which are not) then she will need support whilst she learns how, and should rapidly develop the skill of expressing the milk into a bottle so that someone else can feed the baby at night. Most breastfed babies require feeding every 2 to 3 hours at first. They gain weight initially more slowly than bottle-fed babies. Nowadays, if all has gone well, after a day or two you will be encouraged to go home (you may stay in hospital longer if there have been complications or a Caesarean operation). So, you go home where the stress, the worries, the sleeplessness and the joys begin; we will consider some of the issues of living with a child if you have epilepsy in the next chapter.

## Epilepsy and the outcome of pregnancy

There is no modern evidence to suggest that having epilepsy leads to an increased possibility of an adverse outcome of pregnancy (like prematurity, a low birth weight, a low Apgar score (a measure of a child's condition at birth)) or even an increased risk of stillbirth or perinatal death.

**Table 15.1** Breastfeeding—yes or no?

| Drug | Comments |
|------|----------|
| Acetazolamide | First 4–5 days only |
| Carbamazepine | Safe |
| Clobazam | First 4–5 days only (sleepy infant) |
| Clonazepam | First 4–5 days only (sleepy infant) |
| Diazepam | First 4–5 days only (sleepy infant) |
| Ethosuximide | First 4–5 days only |
| Gabapentin | First 4–5 days only (manufacturers' suggestion) |
| Lacosamide | Not currently recommended |
| Lamotrigine | Safe (NOT if premature delivery) |
| Levetiracetam | Safe (our experience; manufacturers' suggest caution) |
| Oxcarbazepine | First 4–5 days (we think safe beyond this) |
| Phenobarbital | First 4–5 days – then caution (sleepy baby) |
| Phenytoin | First 4–5 days; then manufacturers suggest not |
| Pregabalin | First 4–5 days; otherwise no experience |
| Primidone | As phenobarbital |
| Tiagabine | First 4–5 days but no experience so caution |
| Topiramate | First 4–5 days but not thereafter (abundant in milk) |
| Valproate | Safe |
| Vigabatrin | No exposure best |
| Zonisamide | No exposure best |

Note well: we have been cautious and largely followed the manufacturer's advice (except that for most drugs we have suggested some breastfeeding for at least the first 4–5 days to avoid sudden withdrawal of the infant from the drug, except in those drugs known to be particularly potentially toxic) but, since information changes, do discuss the potential risks of your drug with your consultant. We have occasionally gone beyond the manufacturer's recommendation when Tim has had particular experience of a drug but do remember that if you breastfeed when the manufacturer suggests caution then it will not be held liable if anything goes wrong. It is important to note that this advice relates to those patients taking a single drug; for those taking two or more the risk of an adverse event is clearly greater.

One or two modern studies suggest that pre-eclampsia is commoner in women with epilepsy than would be expected by chance, although this has certainly not been Tim's experience. It has been reported that children born to mothers taking carbamazepine have a slightly smaller head circumference at birth than children born to mothers not taking carbamazepine (but they catch up quickly and with no difference in birth length or placental weight) and that there is an increase in fetal distress in children born to mothers taking valproate, but, again, this has not been Tim's experience.

Haemorrhagic disease of the newborn can be prevented by prescribing vitamin K (see Chapter 7). Careful monitoring of women with epilepsy whilst pregnant, and preventing seizures by judicious increases of their medication, seems to be important in preventing obstetric complications. It is important to remember that those few studies that have looked at the pregnancy outcomes of women with uncontrolled epilepsy and not taking anticonvulsant medication have a far higher fetal abnormality rate than even the old uncontrolled studies of pregnancy outcome in women taking anticonvulsants.

## The partner's role (support, support, support)

Your role as partner to the person giving birth is often unsung and unhonoured but, nevertheless, vital. Make sure your partner gets enough sleep by helping with the night feeding (whether expressed breast milk or bottle) and put aside your own fatigue to make sure you are there when needed.

Be prepared to adapt your day and its tasks to help her and support her through the first few days of tears and despair (this is quite normal; the pain of childbirth soon fades). Interestingly, possibly because many anticonvulsants are also antidepressants, the incidence, in Tim's experience, of depression in women with epilepsy is actually quite low but be on the lookout for sustained low mood or despair and report it quickly to your doctor.

Your role is to share the joys and support the lows of new childhood. In particular, if you have to go back to work make sure that your partner has support from elsewhere, knows how to change and take the baby out safely, but does not bath the baby on her own (see Chapter 16). Soon, together, you will have got the hang of things, realised what you have let yourselves in for, and may even start thinking about the next one (see Chapter 11 on contraception, you mad fools); if necessary help her sort out her epilepsy more before embarking on the next addition to your family.

One other thing; your partner's medication may have been increased during the pregnancy, sometimes by a great deal. Shortly after the birth the dose will have to drop again, so you and your partner should follow the instructions given about reduction and know the warning signs of intoxication (unsteadiness, dizziness, double vision, and drunkenness; fatigue, remember, is part and parcel of having a new baby!) and be prepared to drop the dose if and when these symptoms appear; you will often find that the eventual dose she ends up on is slightly higher than the one she started out on, but this does not matter since early childhood is tiring and stressful and seizures therefore more likely.

# 16

# Childcare if you have epilepsy

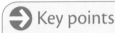

## Key points

- Make sure, whatever the distractions, that you take your medication on time.
- Make sure you have the right priorities (keep the baby clean, rather than the piano).
- Mood swings are normal in the first week or two (nothing to do with the epilepsy).
- Get enough sleep (if breastfeeding, express enough for your partner to do night feeds).
- Make kitchens especially (but everywhere) childproof and safe.
- Teach child from the age of 2 years what to do if you have a seizure (i.e. stay with you).
- Teach child from about the age of 3 years how to summon help.

## So, what is important, what's not?

Before your partner goes back to work sort out what is important and what is not. You are the most important; you, your baby and, of course, your epilepsy.

Firstly, take your medicine regularly and properly, no matter what distractions surround you. Then decide which household tasks are essential (or can be made your partner's responsibility) and which can be left. So you didn't dust the lounge today (or yesterday)? Big deal! (And what are partners for?). Is the baby in reasonably clean clothes? Has she been fed? Is she sleeping peacefully? She is? Great—you are doing better than most, and you with your epilepsy.

Do remember, in particular, that swings of mood between joyful (if slightly manic) laughter and deep tearful despair is normal for the first week or so after birth, which has nothing to do with you or your epilepsy but everything to do with the hormonal changes taking place as your body adjusts to no longer having a baby inside it. These mood swings will pass and don't need treating (but do need an understanding partner).

The most important thing for you is to get enough sleep, which, as we have already said, is where your partner comes in. And those relatives and friends that come crowding through the door to see and play with your little miracle? Put them to work! They can help with the washing up, and the ironing (what are mothers and mothers-in-law for, after all?) and it is a small price to pay for being able to see and play with your beautiful baby whilst you get some rest. Listen to the advice that will come pouring into your ears but make sure that you and your partner make the decisions.

# The practical advice

First of all, and most important, any precautions you take should be related to **you** and **your** epilepsy and its risks; it would be all too easy for some 'jobs-worth' to draw up a list of imagined 'precautions' that would deprive you of practically any contact with your baby particularly if there is some granny or social-worker-like figure in the background waiting to take over. Your baby needs you. But, there are some precautions that you should take, irrespective of whether you are still having seizures or not. For, in the first year or so after the birth there is always the risk, even though slight, that they may return because motherhood is tiring and stressful.

# Precautions you should take

What follows is a list of possible precautions. We say possible, because what you do will depend upon you, your circumstances and your epilepsy—and every mother should follow some of them, whether she has epilepsy or not. This list assumes you are on your own in the daytime; if you are not then (a) you lucky so-and-so and (b) make sure you do your share, even if supervised.

### Taking care of baby

- Feed child on floor or sitting against wall if on your own, until she is old enough for a chair.
- Change child on floor or secure bed from which she cannot roll off, if on your own.
- When older always feed her in a secure high chair if on your own with her.
- Never, no matter how dirty (you or the child), bath her on her own.
- Never take the child into the bath with you, unless properly accompanied.

### Transporting baby

- Carry the child in a secure carrycot up and down stairs (never in your arms).
- Use a 'dead man's handle' on pram, so it stops if you fall or wander away.

- Contain crawling, toddling, and walking by safety gates and harnesses (good luck!).
- Use secure reins on your walking child, attached to you (not just in your hand).

---

## Calling all partners!

All partners of women with epilepsy, even if you are currently seizure free, must be prepared to help, something they do not always instinctively understand (they are mostly men, after all!). Do remember that your partner has also had a sudden life change from being the absolute pinnacle of your love and affection to having to share it with a squalling little monster in a cot that suddenly has become the sole focus of your attention; so give him some time and affection as well and he might even vacuum the front room.

---

### Sleeping, feeding, and changing

Sleep is important for all mothers but particularly for you to prevent your epilepsy breaking through. Make sure your partner does her or his share at night so that you can sleep properly (this may mean sleeping in a separate room for a while so that the baby's cries wake them and not you and, if breastfeeding, express enough into bottles so that your partner and baby don't have to disturb you.

- Do remember that breastfed babies need feeding every 2–3 hours at first so you may need to express more than you think.
- Try not to mix breast and bottle until breastfeeding is fully established, unless you are trying to disengage from the breast.
- Don't feel defeated if you have to switch; many people have to in our present society which isn't really geared up for the exclusive care that young children actually need.

When you are feeding your child, whether from breast or bottle, do it on the floor; that is, sit with your back against a wall and the baby on your arm or in your lap—sit on a clean cloth or towel if you want to. This way, if you do have a seizure you have very little chance of harming the baby as she cannot drop or be crushed by the weight of your body (and, if you do feel a seizure coming on put the baby into a place of safety—a clean floor will do). If you are likely to have frequent seizures it is probably best if there is always someone with you when you feed your child, but make sure you still do it and don't become a passive spectator watching someone else feed **your** child.

Likewise when you are changing or dressing your child do it on the floor on a clean towel or cloth; that way if you have a seizure there is no bed or changing trolley for the child to roll off. When the child is old enough feed her, properly fastened, in a sturdy 'high chair' so that, if you were to have a seizure she would remain secure in the chair. The more secure and less anxious you feel about handling your child the less likely you are to have a seizure.

## Bathing

It is important that you do not bath your child on your own, no matter how smelly the provocation, but always have someone with you. Never take the child into the bath with you when you have one unless, again, you have someone with you (remember we said in an earlier chapter to have someone with you when you bathe anyway). We do know of a mother who bathed alone with her baby, had a seizure and very nearly drowned with her child (and she had been seizure free for 7 years—but her chemist had just changed her brand of anticonvulsant).

## Moving baby

Until it can walk, with you holding its hand, carry the child up and down stairs secure in a carrycot, never in your arms (we know of a girl who dropped her baby in a seizure on the stairs).

Before you know it your currently passive little baby will discover the joys of crawling then walking and will be off down the garden or up the stairs quick as lightning (yes, grandson Harry, you may only be 2 but Tim means you, 'Flash Harry' indeed!).

Sit down with your partner and work out how best to make your dwelling into a 'safe house' where, if you are alone with your child and have a seizure, she or he will remain with you and not wander away upstairs or out into the garden or down the front path and while remaining with you will not tip hot water over or eat something disagreeable. This will require some thought and a little expense (for safety gates, harnesses etcetera) but is well worth doing. The kitchen is potentially the most dangerous place, for both you and your child (even if you don't have a seizure). Epilepsy Action (which used to be the British Epilepsy Association) or your own national epilepsy association can help with advice.

## When you go out

- Make sure that there is a 'dead man's handle' device on the pram or push-chair so that if you lose your grip it will stop with you (good pram shops can advise).

- Try to cross the road using a proper pedestrian crossing (where the traffic has to stop for as long as you are on it) rather than a light controlled one, which barely gives time enough for the nimble to cross, or use an underpass; this may mean planning your journey carefully.

◆ If you are prone to frequent seizures then encourage one of your neighbours or relatives to go with you, making sure that they know what to do if you have a seizure.

◆ When your child will no longer go in the pram (by age 1 if she is anything like granddaughter Isabella) but insists on walking then make sure she is on reins which are attached to you (rather than just in your hand) so that if you do lose awareness the child remains fastened securely to you until you recover and doesn't wander off; this is particularly important in traffic or by water.

## Teaching your child about epilepsy

◆ By about the age of 2 the child should be taught to remain with you if you have a seizure.

◆ By 3 may well be able to summon help.

◆ By 5 or 6 the child should know what to do if you have a seizure (remember that emphatic child we told you about earlier? Yes, that one, the one that said 'bugger off—I'm in charge!'). Make sure she or he knows what to do if you should have a seizure but don't drag the poor little person everywhere with you just in case you have a seizure; let her or him live a little. Take a friend instead if you can, sometimes.

Finally, as an addendum, we (an epilepsy nurse and Tim) considered the outcome of epilepsy in two groups of patients in the first 12 months after the birth of their child:

The first group of 187 patients (57 of whom had a seizure during this period in their lives) were women seen in our preconception clinic and epilepsy and pregnancy clinic and followed up afterwards for at least 12 months. All had had counselling and/or a home visit after the birth from our nurse practitioner (who herself had epilepsy) with a full discussion of precautions to be taken as outlined above.

The other group of 38 women, all with active epilepsy, were referred to our clinic for the first time in the 12 months after the birth of their child, only 2 of whom had had any kind of safety counselling.

The two groups were obviously, therefore, not directly comparable but it is interesting that in the first group only 3 minor safety incidents occurred (1 in 60 or 1 in 20 of those with active epilepsy) whilst in the second group 12 incidents occurred (3 in 10) of which 8 were serious (potentially life threatening to the baby, 2 in 10). Safety counselling seemed therefore to have some value.

# 17

# The menopause and epilepsy

> ## → Key points
>
> - A premature menopause may be slightly more common in women with epilepsy.
> - Epilepsy is likely to start in the menopause more commonly than expected by chance.
> - Women with epilepsy should consider the pros and cons of HRT carefully and should **always** take progesterone as well as oestrogen if they use HRT.
> - They should avoid having their ovaries removed if premenstrual unless essential.
> - Some anticonvulsants are better avoided during and after the menopause.

## The cycle stops and menopause begins

Eventually the menstrual cycle stops and the menopause begins. This is usually between the ages of 45–55, and may be abrupt or the cycle may just peter out. In the UK, the oldest woman to have had a natural pregnancy was 58 when, much to her and her partner's surprise, she conceived.

A premature menopause (aged 35 or under) is possibly more common in women with epilepsy, probably because of the effect that epilepsy can have on the smooth running of the menstrual cycle, which is why we suggest having your first child by the age of 30 if you have epilepsy. However, we do know of women with epilepsy having their first (and subsequent) children in their 40s.

## Medics usually divide the stages of the menopause into three:

- ◆ *The premenopause* starts at the age of 30 with a slight loss of body calcium. This loss continues slowly until the menopause at which point it accelerates to a rate of about 5% per year for the next 5 years or so before declining again.

- ◆ *The perimenopause* starts at 35 when relative fertility declines. Periods may become heavier and more irregular (not if you are using hormonal contraception).

- ◆ *The menopause* starts usually between 45–55 with cessation of the periods. It is usually advised, unless the menopause has been caused by hysterectomy, to continue with contraception for a couple of years after menstruation has apparently stopped in case the ovaries unexpectedly squeeze out one or two more eggs (it has happened).

At the menopause the woman may have to endure unpleasant symptoms of hot flushes, night sweats and depression. Why some women get these symptoms severely and others hardly at all is unknown, but they can be a real nuisance, both to the woman herself and to her family, although they eventually subside and disappear.

## Will epilepsy get better or worse (or even start)?

Women with true premenstrual epilepsy (using the narrower medical definition) may have a worsening or re-awakening of their seizures during the perimenopause but, once the menopause has been fully reached, they usually disappear. However, during the menopause a few previously quiescent epilepsies may restart despite continued medication (see Case study of Annie, Chapter 5) or, if established, may become more intense or change the nature of their presentation (see Case study of Jennifer, this chapter).

The menopause is a time of hormonal and emotional changes, which can sometimes precipitate or worsen epilepsy. Epilepsy is probably slightly more likely to start in the menopause than would be expected by chance. If it does occur it is important to get it under control quickly (Tim has known several sad occurrences of sudden death in epilepsy occurring at this time). Because of the possible need for HRT and other drugs (like those to control blood pressure) it is best to use epilepsy medication that is not enzyme inducing. How much HRT is itself responsible for the supposed 40% increase in seizure frequency in women with epilepsy at this time is currently unclear, but the use of HRT should be approached with caution by women with epilepsy.

# Hormone replacement therapy

Oestrogen, the main hormone used in HRT, is certainly proconvulsant (increases the risk of seizures) and if you have epilepsy should almost always be used in conjunction with progesterone, which is also used in HRT, but not always. If a woman in the menopause using HRT still has her womb then it is usual to use both oestrogen and progesterone in the medication (a bit like the combined oral contraceptive) because oestrogen on its own can cause endometrial hyperplasia (overgrowth of the lining of the womb), which can lead to cancer. The perceived disadvantage of this for some women is that regular episodes of uterine blood loss (akin to a period) will continue for as long as the mixture is taken.

If the woman has lost her womb through surgery then the progesterone is not needed and oestrogen is given on its own (it is thought that the addition of progesterone may increase the side effect risk of HRT). But, if you have epilepsy you should continue to take progesterone with the oestrogen regardless, partly because the latter on its own is convulsant, and partly because progesterone has probable anticonvulsant properties (indeed it has been tried as an anticonvulsant, but only in men).

It can be difficult to persuade those doctors who prescribe HRT that a woman with epilepsy always needs progesterone regardless of her surgical status, but Tim's experience suggests that it is a worthwhile precaution. Jennifer's case study is an example where unopposed oestrogen can precipitate seizures; it is important to point out that neither Jennifer nor her doctors realised that she had epilepsy, and oestrogen HRT is the recognized treatment of an acute menopause caused by surgical removal of the uterus and ovaries.

# Maybe leave the ovaries behind (if still having periods)

This leads to another problem for the woman with epilepsy. Surgical removal of the uterus (hysterectomy) nowadays is usually accompanied by removal of the ovaries because of the small but real risk of ovarian cancer if they are left behind. This leads to an acute menopause for which some form of HRT is needed. If the woman has epilepsy it may be better, if she is still having periods, to leave the ovaries behind and allow a natural menopause to occur later; this is obviously not possible if there is already pathology in the ovaries. Again, discuss this with the person doing the operation who may need some persuading!

# HRT or not, if you have epilepsy?

- If you can do without HRT, then do so.
- If you do need to commence HRT, take the combination of oestrogen and progesterone.
- Modern practice suggests taking it for no more than about 5 years.

- ◆ To make sure that you are taking enough progesterone it may be better to use the tablet form rather than patches (although this may slightly increase the risk of an untoward thrombosis (blood clot).

- ◆ Remember that if you are taking enzyme-inducing anticonvulsant medication (carbamazepine, oxcarbazepine, phenobarbital, phenytoin, primidone, topiramate, and zonisamide) then you may need to take more HRT than usual to counter the medication's effects on the blood level; this is something to discuss with your medical advisor.

## The importance of calcium

From before the menopause starts there is a slow but steady loss of calcium from the bones, which accelerates for about 5 years when the menopause is reached, before declining again. Some of this loss is unavoidable but can be partly circumvented by:

- ◆ Making sure there is enough calcium and vitamin D in your diet to counteract it. You should be taking at least 1500 milligrams of calcium a day and 400 units of vitamin D. Consult with your doctor or nurse about whether there is enough in your diet or whether you should be taking supplements.

- ◆ Some anticonvulsant drugs (phenobarbital, phenytoin, and primidone in particular, though any enzyme-inducing drug could be at risk) may lead to an increased risk of osteoporosis (softening of the bones) and calcium supplementation may be particularly necessary.

- ◆ Phenytoin may have other effects on calcium metabolism and is probably best avoided.

- ◆ HRT may slow down or obviate menopausal related loss of calcium, which is one of the main reasons for using it.

Other medicines are now used around the menopause to prevent some of its effects. Testosterone (the male hormone) is sometimes used (and may spice up a flagging sexual drive). It is quite safe if you have epilepsy, as are tibolone and tamoxifen (but, if you are taking valproate it is worthwhile having your platelet count checked occasionally and blood levels of liver-metabolized anticonvulsants measured if you are taking tamoxifen).

Until more research is done, approach the use of biphosphonates and teriparatide with caution and discuss the pros and cons with your medical and nursing advisor. At the time of writing this book there is no evidence, but after this book is published there may well be more information, which your advisor can access for you.

# 📄 Case study

**Jennifer** was 49, married with three children and had been in good health when she entered an acute menopause. Her periods had been heavy and overfrequent for a couple of years so she had a hysterectomy and bilateral ovariectomy (removal of womb and both ovaries). She recovered from the operation quickly and started on an oral oestrogen HRT (normal practice).

Three months later she had an episode of 'feeling strange and out of this world' followed by a 30-second loss of consciousness, in which she remained standing, recovering very quickly. Two days later the same odd feeling occurred but this time followed by a brief tonic clonic seizure (witnessed by a friend who was with her).

An EEG showed clear-cut epileptic activity and an MRI of her head showed an obvious and long-standing left hippocampal sclerosis. It was suggested that she stop her HRT at once and start a small dose of lamotrigine. She had no more seizures and her EEG returned to normal. She has chosen to remain on lamotrigine because she wanted to drive again as soon as possible and has continued in her previous employment.

It is impossible to prove but it was suggested that she had had the hippocampal atrophy for some considerable time and this had been awakened into epileptic activity by the convulsant effect of the oestrogen in her HRT unopposed by any progesterone. She also admitted that for as long as she could remember she had had odd brief feelings of detachment, particularly when tired or premenstrual, to which she had paid no attention as she assumed that 'everybody gets them'. Since taking lamotrigine she has had no more.

# 18

# The older woman and epilepsy

## Key points

◆ New onset epilepsy is as common in those aged over 65 as it is under the age of 15 because as the brain ages it acquires scars and injuries.

◆ Older people with epilepsy are less steady on their feet and deficient in calcium so can fall and fracture easily.

◆ Epilepsy in the elderly is often easy to treat, even if associated with strokes or dementia.

◆ Kidney and liver function should be checked prior to the prescription of medication.

◆ Once the epilepsy is under control the person can continue to live independently.

## Women live longer than men

In terms of epilepsy at least, men and women become more similar with age but there remains one important difference: women live longer than men and are therefore more exposed to the ills and trials of old age which can sometimes cause epilepsy. There is no doubt that new-onset epilepsy is as common after the age of 65 as it is under 15 although the causes are different. Sometimes a childhood injury to the brain may not declare itself as epilepsy until much later in life. As the brain ages it may acquire damage, which can pass unrecognized until it becomes a focus for epilepsy. As in Audrey's experience (see Case study, this chapter), elderly people who develop epilepsy are often not properly investigated; the epilepsy and any intellectual deterioration being wrongly put down as an inevitable consequence of old age.

## Added complications

◆ Older people may suffer from unnecessary stigma related to epilepsy, since their ideas about and knowledge of epilepsy may have been formed when prejudice about epilepsy was more widespread and more severe.

- They are also less steady on their feet with weaker skeletons so are more likely to fracture their bones if they fall in a seizure.
- They are also more likely to suffer side effects from anticonvulsant medication.
- Epilepsy, unless rapidly controlled, may also prevent an older person from continuing to live on her or his own (see Mary's case study, this chapter).

These are all good reasons to swiftly investigate and control epilepsy occurring in people over the age of 65. Sadly, this is often not done, with the epilepsy being diagnosed as something else or ignored because some other disorder like dementia is apparently present. About 10% of people with Alzheimer's disease and atherosclerotic dementia will develop concomitant epilepsy, which, particularly if simple or complex partial seizures, may pass unnoticed and untreated.

## It's not all gloom

> Epilepsy occurring for the first time in old age, even if it is the accompaniment of some other bodily or brain disorder, is usually comparatively easy to treat, often with a relatively small amount of medication.

It is best to choose, for new onset seizures, medication that is not enzyme inducing. A low slow-dose increase is also best in the elderly. It is most important, before starting any anticonvulsant treatment in an elderly person, to ensure that both kidneys and liver are working satisfactorily; if either is not then careful dose adjustments will have to be made (and seizures can be a symptom of rapid kidney failure). If there is a brain or bodily cause of the seizures, that may need treating as well, for instance, raised blood pressure.

Although we have chosen Audrey as an example of an older person with a long-standing (if initially unrecognized) primary brain tumour, many brain tumours in old age, whether they cause epileptic seizures or not, are secondary; that is they have spread from a primary tumour elsewhere in the body, like the breast or lung. Although this is obviously very serious and potentially fatal, nowadays it need not be; the primary tumour can be removed surgically and the secondary tumour sometimes as well, or controlled with chemotherapy or radiotherapy.

It is important to remember that not everyone with a definable brain lesion will necessarily develop epilepsy; other factors, probably mainly genetic, are involved as well. The need for adequate calcium and vitamin D in the diet remains important.

## Epilepsy that persists into old age

It is important to review epilepsy carefully. Is it really epilepsy? If it is, has it been fully investigated in case there is a definable and treatable cause? Are there treatments that have not been tried? It is worth doing this and not just leaving old people on the same medication that they have been taking for the past 40 years. People with epilepsy in old age need just as much care and medical consideration as younger people. And that takes us back to where we started; as these last two case studies illustrate—never give up, never stop trying. Live your life, as we shall see in the last chapter.

 Case study

**Mary** was 68 and was a retired seamstress. A year before being seen in the clinic she had had a week of feeling a little confused and 'out of sorts' and had some minimal left arm weakness and tingling for a couple of days, all of which passed completely. Her GP diagnosed a mild stroke in the right side of her brain. A few months later she began to have attacks (about 2 or 3 a month) in which she would become confused, disorientated and have left arm tingling; attacks would last some 2–3 minutes although she would then be tired and a little confused for some hours afterwards. Attacks usually occurred in the early morning, between waking and getting up.

She was referred to her local neurology clinic where a CT scan and EEG were reported as normal. It was decided that she was suffering from recurrent transient ischaemic attacks (brief alterations in blood flow in the brain) and she was returned to the care of her GP with the suggestion that her blood pressure was monitored regularly.

She lived on her own and the attacks were therefore potentially dangerous and disabling; she had already had one in the kitchen and her family were keen for her to go into sheltered accommodation, an idea which she resisted. She suggested a second opinion, which the GP agreed to.

A 24-hour EEG showed a clear-cut right temporal spike wave abnormality in the early morning both before and after waking and an MRI scan of her head showed two small right temporal scars. It was suggested that the diagnosis was partial epilepsy consequent upon a previous cerebrovascular accident. Lamotrigine was started at a dose of 5 milligrams a day and slowly escalated. At 50 milligrams a day the seizures stopped and have not returned. Three years later she continues to live in her own home and is slowly adding to her tally of great grandchildren.

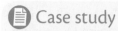 Case study

**Audrey** was born during the First World War. She did very well educationally, and qualified as a doctor in 1938. She married a fellow student and they had one child before he was killed in the Western Desert in 1942.

She never remarried but devoted herself to caring for her daughter and to her career in public health. When she was 63 she made an unfortunate but costly mistake in her work and was advised to retire. It was noted that, previously meticulous in all things, she had become slapdash in her dress and behaviour, her house became somewhat dirty and she failed to remember to pay bills so she moved in with her daughter and her family. Her intellect continued to deteriorate and she became spiteful, with bursts of unreasonable and unprovoked anger. She also became incontinent; sometimes, before being incontinent, she would suddenly lose consciousness for perhaps 30 seconds and loudly smack her lips. The family GP suggested that she would be best managed in his local care home that specialised in what was obviously Alzheimer's' disease.

The daughter asked a nearby specialist epilepsy clinic for help (the clinic had looked after one of the daughter's children). The consultant went to see her and her daughter at home. Audrey could not speak and seemed oblivious to his presence. An ophthalmoscope revealed swelling of both optic nerves suggesting that the diagnosis was not what the GP had thought.

After her admission to a psychogeriatric unit where the seizures responded quickly to carbamazepine, an MRI scan revealed a benign brain tumour that was successfully removed. She returned, somewhat frail, to live in the bosom of her family. About 3 years after the operation, still seizure free, she died peacefully in her sleep.

# 19

# Being a woman, having epilepsy: Harriet's story

This final chapter addresses the practicalities of being a woman with epilepsy. Being such a woman I know that it is not straightforward; many conflicting factors are always present.

I came to terms with epilepsy very quickly as I was only a child and didn't really understand all the problems that epilepsy in an adult would bring. It was not until I considered writing this book, and after some research, that I became fully aware of the complexities of epilepsy and the effect it has on people's lives. I am certainly still no expert. After 14 years of living a happy and fun-filled life with epilepsy I have accepted it as a part of who I am, no matter how irritating it can be. It does not stop me doing things I want to do and, apart from continually trying to find the correct drug and dose, and trying to keep up to date with current issues with epilepsy there is, at the bottom of it all, nothing I can do. Even though at times it can be very frightening and frustrating, I am a woman, I have epilepsy, and I live and enjoy my life. Here is my story so far.

I was diagnosed with epilepsy at the age of 9. I began to have attacks of recurrent stiffness and jerking of my right leg, in clear consciousness. I remember thinking it was 'the man under the bed' coming to get me, especially when I awoke to feel a hand on my throat—my own of course but it had become numb. Apart from this I can't remember the start of my epilepsy. My close friend then, and still now, says she remembers my leg jerking under the desk at school and the teacher not believing me, and only allowing me to go home after crying uncontrollably in what I imagine was confusion. Since then my fits have become easier to describe; they often rouse me out of sleep at night and have occurred in the past during the daytime. Sometimes they are transient and mild but sometimes more severe, in which case my right arm becomes involved as well. A 'shooting' feeling travels down my right leg, which then suddenly stiffens, then relaxes, tenses again, and then relaxes, with the muscle spasms making it difficult to breathe until the attack is over and I am left out of breath. After more severe attacks my leg (and sometimes my arm) is numb and I have a brief inability to bear weight. I often know when I am going to have an attack at night, as I feel unsteady during the day, a feeling that is difficult to describe accurately!

When I first had an attack I saw a local paediatrician who made a diagnosis of 'benign rolandic epilepsy' (motor epilepsy). An EEG at that time was said to show some left-sided spike wave activity (unfortunately both record and report seem to have been subsequently lost). A CT scan was normal. I started on carbamazepine and for a short time the attacks seemed to come under control, but then returned despite my taking larger doses of the drug, which made me feel tired. Valproate was therefore added to my original medication, but this seemed to have no effect on the attacks and made me even more tired. My periods started, but the seizures initially seemed to have no relationship to them (this is no longer the case as there now does seem to be a close but not exact relationship between my periods and my seizures; the reason for this is probably that the full hormonal impact of the menstrual cycle may not appear for some years after it starts).

At this point I saw a visiting paediatric neurologist who initially confirmed the diagnosis of epilepsy (although it clearly was not benign rolandic). He withdrew the sodium valproate and substituted vigabatrin and made some more investigations. A sleep-deprived EEG showed some right-sided slow activity suggestive of epilepsy (but was apparently on the wrong side of my brain since I have right-sided seizures) but did not record any attacks and a low power MRI scan was normal. At this point the neurologist began to doubt the diagnosis of epilepsy and to favour a diagnosis of paroxysmal movement disorder and tried to withdraw the vigabatrin; by this time, too, the effect of vigabatrin on visual fields had become known but luckily my fields, when tested, were normal. Vigabatrin withdrawal was tricky and initially led to increased seizure activity but was finally accomplished. Throughout this time my parents (and myself as I got older and understood more about my condition) became more and more frustrated with the length of time between consultations and the number of different consultants and drugs. The fact that most treatments of epilepsy are trial and error is a hideous feeling, especially when the trial usually leads to error, but one must keep trying. It was the last straw for my parents when I became old enough to be seen by an adult neurologist and the waiting time was going to be 9 months. I know this is a common story for people with epilepsy as it is, in the UK at least, a very under-resourced condition with little medical interest in it, although this is not necessarily so in other countries. Consequently my GP referred me to a specialist epilepsy unit, with my uncertain diagnosis, where I had a 'one-stop' examination (EEG, high power MRI scan of my head and a thorough physical and mental assessment) at the first visit.

I am the sort of person who plans ahead. This doesn't combine well with the treatment of my epilepsy but is good for me as a person; I plan ahead possibly because I have epilepsy, I am persistent and very determined. At 17 I planned to start driving, have a gap year teaching in Africa and travel the world, then go to university to be a teacher, three things that are not very easy for a person with uncontrolled epilepsy. The clinic saw the need to diagnose my epilepsy for my health and so that I could fulfil these ambitions.

My initial 'one-stop' investigation revealed a normal physical screen, normal routine blood tests, normal EEG, and a normal high power MRI (as had every other test so far). The given history of the attacks sounded more like epilepsy than a movement disorder to Tim, my new consultant, but doubts remained particularly in the face of normal investigations; carbamazepine, which so far seemed to be the most successful drug to control my attacks, is also effective in other neurological conditions. It was also clear that this was, in Tim's own words, 'a real teenager's epilepsy' (if it was epilepsy) because it was clearly made worse by lack of sleep, stress, and missed medication. What was also clear was that lowering the dose of carbamazepine made my attacks more frequent and more intense so that any change in medication would have to be made slowly and carefully particularly because I was allegedly a bright teenager, doing well at school, with my plans of travel going full steam ahead. I was also keen to know more about my condition. It was, indeed, partly my travel plans and experiences that made the unit realise the need to set up an email contact service for its patients travelling abroad, and eventually to be able to give guidance and support before, during, and after foreign travel.

So, the first thing to do was to try to sharpen up the diagnosis: this meant overnight video EEG monitoring, but there was a catch. This was something the unit could only do for 2 days and nights and it had no other in-patient resources to fall back on if seizures became too frequent or uncontrollable. It chose not to withdraw medication before monitoring in the way that some units can—although medication withdrawal can create its own problems in terms of diagnosis if seizures occur and one needs to be certain that they are the seizures that the patient normally has.

In the first monitoring session a couple of very minor seizures occurred; observation of them on video was unhelpful (because they were so brief and fragmentary) and the EEG was full of movement artefact and unreadable. A second recording session was arranged and, with some trepidation, anticonvulsant doses were halved for a couple of days and I was partly sleep deprived. This resulted in a bigger seizure (which looked epileptic to the observers) and there were some EEG changes (difficult to read because of artefact again), which did seem to show some left-sided epileptic activity during the seizure. It was decided that epilepsy was probably the correct diagnosis but still with a small degree of doubt. Further drug treatment was pursued as vigorously as possible (but, again with the proviso that I was studying and going abroad a lot during the summer holidays) so drug changes could not be too rapid.

At 18 I travelled around the Sahara and many other countries, but sought my doctor's advice before I went. I was well equipped with drugs that could help me if I got ill. Since then I have been lucky enough to go abroad each year, and although I had seizures, forgotten tablets, and got sick, my memories are all happy and epilepsy doesn't feature in one. I have always been very open about having epilepsy and let people around me know what to do if I have a seizure;

having to 'pop' pills at 8 o'clock morning and night makes it difficult to hide! But everyone I have met and had relationships with has completely understood, and has judged me by my character alone.

During my time at the clinic I had a daytime seizure just after seeing Tim for a routine check up. For me this was slightly embarrassing as I couldn't stand up or reach for my phone, and seizures are generally upsetting. No one noticed, not even the person sitting next to me. However, during this seizure Tim happened to walk past and witnessed the attack, and what was a common event to me was an illuminating event for him. Several things passed through his mind, he told me later, as he watched the brief but intense seizure, particularly just how difficult it is for someone to accurately describe either their own or someone else's seizure. What he saw was far more intense than he would have expected from the description that I had given him; really severe muscular spasms of both leg and arm, and more than the couple he had thought usually occurred. The post-seizure weakness of my leg was also quite marked and it was a little while before I could stand. This may well have been a 'bigger' seizure than usual although in retrospect I do make light of my seizures when I describe them as I suspect other people do.

What also struck him was the look of terror on my face; some of this may have been due to muscle spasms of the seizure activity itself but some of it, he suspected, was due to someone who normally prided herself on her autonomy and control being suddenly jerked out of it, becoming a spectacle and, temporarily, vulnerable. He was probably right, although I don't like to admit it—but, then, who would? When the seizure was over I rapidly returned to my normal self. Tim felt he had learnt a valuable lesson about the reality of seizures, which underlined the need to get them under control. He told me later something that I had not realised; doctors, apart from videotaped images, which are at least one remove from reality, rarely see seizures but have to rely on other people's descriptions of them.

Since then I have continued to go abroad, continued to plan ahead, and I am now a qualified teacher living in London after having a great time at university and meeting and making many lovely friends. I have also just begun to take driving lessions. Because I am still taking my old friend carbamazepine I have not been able to use a conventional oral contraceptive but have had to rely on progestogen injections, which to me is much better than having to take yet more pills. I now have a new consultant and a 'secure' diagnosis of epilepsy. Although far from wanting a family yet (a bit more travelling and living abroad to do before then) I have started to reduce my untidy bundle of tablets, so far relatively successfully in preparation for the family that I want in the future. I know I will never be fully under control as my seizures seem to have a will of their own, and I think that this is the sad lesson that some women, especially of childbearing age when certain drugs are best avoided, must learn.

Although my story is not complete, nor a success, I am happy. I live each day and am determined to continue to 'work hard and play hard' (in my dad's words). Not that I can take all the credit for this; if it wasn't for my close friends and family I certainly wouldn't be the person I am. I need to thank them for understanding me perfectly, for being there when I need them, for letting me do my own thing, and for never treating me like someone who, because of their epilepsy (a tiny part of the person I am) has to be treated with kid gloves. I wish everyone with epilepsy the same opportunities that I have had. They are possible, and having epilepsy is far from being a tragedy.

Everyone with epilepsy deals with it in his or her own way, either through acceptance or denial. All I say is: don't let it stop you, or your loved ones, enjoying life.

# Appendix 1

# Drugs for epilepsy

## First-line drugs

### Carbamazepine

- Effective for partial onset seizures (with or without secondary generalization).

- Also against primary generalized tonic clonic seizures.

- Ineffective against primary absences and myoclonic seizures.

- It induces it own metabolism: an initial satisfactory dose may have to be increased.

- It has a short half-life (but the Retard formulation extends this, so is to be preferred).

- A blood level of the drug is measured and is useful, particularly in pregnancy.

- It is best to start with a low dose and build up gradually to avoid side effects.

- *Enzyme inducing?*—Yes, strongly; usual dose of 'the pill' not effective.

*Side effects*

- *Dose related*—double vision, unsteadiness, nausea and vomiting, difficulty in concentration, agitation and rash.

- *Hypersensitivity*—rare Stevens–Johnson syndrome (rash, raised temperature, liver and kidney failure, potentially fatal) usually prevented by low slow initial dose increments, low white cell count in the blood (but will usually respond to infection), rare total organ failure.

- *Chronic toxicity*—can cause a low level of sodium in the blood, which can occasionally cause symptoms and needs checking from time to time; can also affect thyroid function tests.

- *Does it affect the unborn baby?*—modern studies suggest that in reasonable monotherapy doses it is unlikely to and is one of the safer drugs. There are unconfirmed reports that children born to mothers taking a high dose at birth may have scholastic difficulties later in life.

- *Pregnancy*—take folic acid 5 milligrams daily by mouth from before pregnancy starts and all the way through and vitamin K 10 milligrams daily by mouth from the 36th week of pregnancy until the end. Measure blood level of carbamazepine before the pregnancy starts and maintain it at that level by judicious dose increases during the pregnancy (see Chapter 14 for the Birmingham experience).

◆ *Breastfeeding*—this seems safe long term (as less than half the blood level present in milk).

## Lamotrigine

◆ A first-line drug for all seizure types.

◆ As with carbamazepine best to start with a low dose and build up slowly.

◆ If used second line, carbamazepine significantly reduces its blood level, valproate significantly raises it.

◆ If starting 'the pill' often best to increase the dose of lamotrigine by a third to a half.

◆ A blood level is measured and is useful, particularly in pregnancy.

◆ It is effective against photo and pattern sensitivity.

◆ *Enzyme inducing?*—No

### Side effects

◆ *Dose related*—unsteadiness, double vision, vomiting, and rash.

◆ *Hypersensitivity*—rare Stevens–Johnson syndrome (rash, raised temperature, liver and kidney failure, potentially fatal) usually prevented by low slow initial dose increments.

◆ *Chronic toxicity*—a rare lupus-like syndrome has been reported.

◆ *Does it affect the unborn baby?*—As with carbamazepine reasonably safe in pregnancy (though caution in monotherapy doses much over 200 milligrams a day).

◆ *Pregnancy*—take folic acid 5 milligrams daily by mouth from before the pregnancy starts and all the way through. Measure the blood level of lamotrigine monthly and increase the dose to maintain the same blood level (see Chapter 14). Reduce the dose when the pregnancy is over.

◆ *Breastfeeding*—safe if the child is at term (breast milk contains about 50% of the blood level) **but do not breastfeed if child is premature** as she will not be able to metabolize it.

## Levetiracetam

◆ It is powerful and has a wide spectrum of action against all seizure types.

◆ Very effective against photo and pattern sensitivity.

◆ It can be given in a therapeutic dose from the outset if required.

◆ Care is needed in patients with renal failure.

- Blood levels are not monitored.
- *Enzyme inducing?*—No.

*Side effects*

- *Dose related*—nausea, difficulty in sleeping, weight changes.
- *Hypersensitivity*—rare aggression.
- *Chronic toxicity*—none yet reported (but is still comparatively new).
- *Does it affect the unborn baby?*—No convincing evidence that it does in mono-therapy although, as a comparatively new drug, numbers are still small; animal data also does not suggest teratogenicity in doses comparable to the human dose.
- *Pregnancy*—take 5 milligrams of folic acid daily from before the start of the pregnancy and all the way through. Efficacy of a dose increase in pregnancy uncertain.
- *Breastfeeding*—it is almost certainly safe to do so, although numbers are still small.

## Oxcarbazepine

- The spectrum of effectiveness is similar to that of carbamazepine.
- Introduced comparatively recently into the UK but used for much longer elsewhere.
- It would probably be preferable to carbamazepine were it not for the cost.
- *Enzyme inducing?*—Yes, probably less than carbamazepine: care with 'the pill'.

*Side effects*

- *Dose related*—double vision, unsteadiness, nausea and vomiting; as with carbamazepine but probably less often.
- *Hypersensitivity*—severe rash, as with carbamazepine, but possibly less common.
- *Chronic toxicity*—can cause low serum sodium, which can give rise to symptoms of tiredness, vomiting, and diarrhoea (more often than with carbamazepine), so suggest checking serum electrolytes from time to time.
- *Does it affect the unborn baby?*—The data sheet reports cleft palate and neural tube defects but it is not clear if this relates to oxcarbazepine alone and probably the incidence of fetal abnormality (in relatively small monotherapy doses) is low as with carbamazepine. Discuss with your doctor.
- *Pregnancy*—folic acid 5 milligrams daily by mouth should be taken from before a pregnancy commences and all the way through. Vitamin K should be taken, 10 milligrams by mouth daily, from week 36 of the pregnancy as with carbamazepine until delivery. No evidence that the dose has to be increased during pregnancy, but possibly so, as with carbamazepine.

- *Breastfeeding*—breast milk contains about 50% of the maternal blood level of oxcarbazepine and although the manufacturers suggest caution breastfeeding is likely to be as safe as with carbamazepine and certainly should be undertaken for the first 4 or 5 days after birth, and longer if the woman wishes to.

## Second-line drugs

### Gabapentin

- A good second-line drug for partial seizures with or without secondary generalization.
- It has been around long enough that it can be first line except it can be expensive.
- Whether it is useful in primary generalized epilepsy is also unclear.
- Lack of interactions makes it useful, as does its lack of serious side effects.
- Dose can go up rapidly if needed.
- Blood level is not routinely measured.
- *Enzyme inducing?*—No.

*Side effects*

- *Dose related*—nausea and unsteadiness.
- *Hypersensitivity*—sometimes serious aggression.
- *Chronic toxicity*—weight gain.
- *Does it affect the unborn baby?*—No real evidence that it does and 'clean' animal data.
- *Pregnancy*—take folic acid 5 milligrams by mouth daily from before pregnancy and all the way through. No evidence that the dose needs to be increased.
- *Breastfeeding*—suggest some for first 4 or 5 days at least. Manufacturers suggest no breastfeeding but possibly are being ultra cautious; discuss with your specialist.

### Pregabalin

- A new drug, related to, but not the same as, gabapentin.
- For partial onset seizures, with or without secondary generalization.
- As yet there is no evidence about its efficacy in primary generalized seizures.
- Excreted via the kidneys so care in patients with renal failure.
- Blood level monitoring is not done.
- *Enzyme inducing?*—No.

*Side effects*

- *Dose related*—sleepiness, unsteadiness, blurred vision, dry mouth, and weight increase.

- *Hypersensitivity*—should not be taken if you have hereditary disorders of sugar metabolism (consult your doctor and the data sheet).

- *Chronic toxicity*—none yet reported (but it is a new drug).

- *Does it affect the unborn baby?*—No human experience although animal data is clean; take folic acid 5 milligrams by mouth daily from before the pregnancy and all the way through.

- *Pregnancy*—no evidence yet about whether dose increase is needed.

- *Breastfeeding*—no evidence on which to base a decision, although some suggested for 4–5 days after delivery to avoid abrupt withdrawal of the drug in the infant; observe the child carefully.

## Tiagabine

- A second-line drug for partial seizures with or without secondary generalization.

- No evidence about its efficacy in primary generalized epilepsy.

- Blood level not measured.

- *Enzyme inducing?*—No.

*Side effects*

- *Dose related*—sleepiness and unsteadiness; psychosis and depression have been reported.

- *Hypersensitivity*—partial status (see Case study of Samantha, Chapter 2) said to be not uncommon.

- *Chronic toxicity*—there is no evidence (yet) that it causes chronic visual impairment, although it is related to the obsolete anticonvulsant drug vigabatrin, which certainly does (see p. 152).

- *Does it affect the unborn baby?*—Animal data reportedly clean but no human data.

- *Pregnancy*—take 5 milligrams of folic acid daily from before the pregnancy starts and all the way through. No evidence (either way) that dose has to be increased in pregnancy.

- *Breastfeeding*—no evidence available so suggest limiting breastfeeding to the first 4 or 5 days, but discuss with your specialist.

# Third-line drugs

## Clobazam

- This is one of the family of benzodiazepine (tranquillizer) drugs.

- It shares its anticonvulsant properties with many of them.

- Mainly used as a premenstrual drug, for up to 10 days (it can be extremely useful).

- Or as a one-off treatment for seizure clusters where again it is often successful.

- A recent study has shown it is a useful third-line drug in addition to its specialist roles.

- Make sure your doctor knows to write SLS after the drug's name on the prescription.

- Blood levels are not measured.

- *Enzyme inducing?*—No.

### Side effects

- *Dose related*—drowsiness.

- *Hypersensitivity*—disinhibited behaviour, aggression, occasional rash.

- *Chronic toxicity*—possible dependence, this is reasonably unlikely with this particular drug, which has a slightly different formula from other benzodiazepine drugs.

- *Does it affect the unborn baby?*—No real evidence that it does, although manufacturers cautiously suggest not using it in the first trimester of pregnancy but if you are taking it continually you will have to and the risk is probably small; if you have planned the pregnancy and are seizure free on clobazam then it is probably safer to stay on it than to try to come off it. This is something you must discuss with your doctor and reach a joint decision about.

- *Pregnancy*—take 5 milligrams of folic acid daily from before starting the pregnancy and all the way through. Risk of sleepy newborn infant if used to break up a cluster of seizures in labour but this is usually acceptable.

- *Breastfeeding*—apart from the first 4–5 days after birth suggest do not breastfeed as there is a risk of an overly sleepy infant.

### Clonazepam

- This is another benzodiazepine drug related to diazepam.

- Used orally for treating epilepsy and intravenously for treating status epilepticus.

- It is a third-line drug, mainly employed for resistant primary generalized seizures.

- It has a long half-life so is usually taken once a day.

- The effective therapeutic dose and the toxic dose are usually fairly close together.

- It has to be used carefully with concurrent valproate.

- Blood level is not measured.

- *Enzyme inducing?*—No.

*Side effects*

- *Dose related*—drooling (particularly in the learning disabled), irritability, and memory impairment.
- *Hypersensitivity*—aggressive episodes, disinhibition, rare rash.
- *Chronic toxicity*—dependence.
- *Does it affect the unborn baby?*—Very little evidence either way so, as with clobazam, discuss with your doctor.
- *Pregnancy*—take folic acid 5 milligrams daily by mouth from before the start of the pregnancy and all the way through.
- *Breastfeeding*—for no more than 4 or 5 days after delivery to avoid a too sleepy baby.

## Lacosamide

- A new drug currently licenced as 'add on' medication for partial onset seizures (with or without secondary generalization) in patients over the age of 16.
- Does not affect blood levels of carbamazepine or valproate, nor is it affected by them.
- Does not affect blood level of 'the pill' or progesterone.
- Blood level not measured.
- Not enzyme inducing.
- If offered it, discuss pros and cons carefully with your doctor (who must have read the Data Sheet).

## Side effects

- *Dose related*—see Data Sheet; may exacerbate heart conduction problems, so have full ECG read before you take it.
- *Hypersensitivity*—see above.
- *Chronic toxicity*—as yet unknown.
- *Dose it affect the unborn baby?*—Not currently recommended in those wishing to become pregnant as no human experience (though comparatively 'clean' animal data).
- *Pregnancy*—not advised; folic acid 5mgm daily from before the pregnancy if patient does become pregnant.
- *Breastfeeding*—not recommended (particularly as currently taken with at least one other anticonvulsant).

## Topiramate

- A potentially very useful drug for all types of epilepsy, it was introduced too rapidly and with far too high an initial dose.
- This led to many unwanted and serious side effects.
- Now with a small initial dose and escalated slowly the drug is used widely again.

- It is a potential first-line drug but best avoided in women until after the menopause.
- Blood levels not used.
- *Enzyme inducing?*—Certainly in higher doses; discuss risk with your doctor.

### Side effects

- *Dose related*—sleepiness, slowed thinking, weight loss (sometimes severe), schizophrenia-like psychosis (clears if the drug is withdrawn), depressive psychosis (also clears on drug withdrawal), irritating tingling in hands and feet.
- *Hypersensitivity*—an eye disorder (acute short sight with raised eye fluid pressure—glaucoma). Must be recognized quickly to avoid permanent damage so report any change in your vision at once. Usually occurs in the first month of taking the drug.
- *Chronic toxicity*—kidney stones; all patients taking it should make sure that they have a good fluid intake.
- *Does it affect the unborn baby?*—The evidence is fairly compelling that it does, with limb abnormalities reported in animals and hypospadias (an abnormality in the development of the penis) in humans.
- *Pregnancy*—take folic acid 5 milligrams by mouth daily from before the pregnancy starts and all the way through, and vitamin K 10 mgm daily by mouth from the 36th week until the end, but until further evidence is available, suggest if possible avoiding this drug if you are a woman who definitely wants, at some stage, to become pregnant. No evidence that dose has to be increased in pregnancy.
- Breastfeeding—found in abundance in breast milk so data sheet suggests not to breastfeed, but some breastfeeding for the first 4 or 5 days only to avoid precipitate withdrawal of the drug from the infant, but not thereafter, is probably important.

### Valproate

- First line for all epilepsies (and photic and pattern sensitivity).
- But not in women before the menopause (as can affect the unborn baby).
- A blood level is quoted but little used clinically.
- Blood levels of lamotrigine are much higher than expected if taken with valproate.
- Increases the amount of active phenytoin so its blood levels are misleading.
- *Enzyme inducing?*—No (but is enzyme inhibiting if taken with lamotrigine).

### Side effects

- *Dose related*—shaking hands, weight gain, and irritability.

◆ *Hypersensitivity*—liver failure (this is mainly in infants and young children) and inflammation of the pancreas (both can be fatal unless recognized early).

◆ *Chronic toxicity*—hair loss (rarely complete), menstrual irregularity (or cessation) and the polycystic ovary syndrome (see Chapter 9).

◆ *Does it affect the unborn baby?*—Definitely: defects reported include spina bifida (maldevelopment of the lower spinal cord), a specific facial abnormality, abnormalities of skeletal and limb development, heart defects, and hypospadias (abnormality in the development of the penis). In large doses, may cause a lowering of intelligence in children of mothers who took it during pregnancy. Coupled with its effect on ovarian function a drug that women, from early adolescence to the menopause, should avoid if at all possible.

◆ *Pregnancy*—if it has to be taken before and during pregnancy (as it sometimes is) then the woman and her partner should be counselled and informed of the various abnormalities that may occur, with careful scans of the child's intra-uterine development, and the dose converted to 3–4 times a day to try to avoid high peaks in blood levels. She should take folic acid 5 milligrams by mouth daily from before the pregnancy starts and throughout it. Some authorities say that a dose of valproate of less than one gram a day is safe, but in the Birmingham University Seizure Clinic spina bifida has been seen in a child of a mother taking only 400 milligrams a day.

◆ *Breastfeeding*—only a little valproate gets into breast milk so breastfeeding need not be restricted.

## Zonisamide

◆ A new drug for patients with partial onset seizures and secondary generalization.

◆ Not for women who may become pregnant.

◆ Prescribers are urged to read the data sheet before writing the first prescription.

◆ Blood levels are not measured.

◆ *Enzyme inducing?*—Yes although manufacturers suggest this is of little practical importance. However, other enzyme-inducing drugs (such as carbamazepine) significantly reduce the amount of zonisamide in the blood stream.

### Side effects

◆ *Dose related*—rash, fatigue, word-finding difficulty, and mental slowing.

◆ *Hypersensitivity*—must not be given to any patient who is hypersensitive to sulphonamide drugs (see data sheet).

◆ *Chronic toxicity*—aplastic anaemia and very low white cell count (drug must be stopped immediately), psychosis (severe mental illness) and depression, and kidney stones (ensure a good fluid intake).

◆ *Does it affect the unborn baby?*—Yes in several animal species at comparatively low dose so must assume the same applies in humans at least until clear evidence is available.

◆ *Pregnancy*—should be avoided in women of child-bearing potential if at all possible but, if it cannot, be then take folic acid 5 milligrams daily from before the pregnancy starts and all the way through it (no evidence that this will be protective against fetal abnormality in this drug) plus vitamin K 10 milligrams by mouth daily from the 36th week of the pregnancy until the end).

◆ *Breastfeeding*—suggest avoid completely, even for the first few days, as there is concern that the drug may be toxic in the newborn. Discuss this with your specialist as further information becomes available.

## Special use drugs

### Acetazolamide

◆ This is a diuretic (water excreting) drug used in premenstrual seizures also used in treating some forms of glaucoma (an eye disorder).

◆ It is used intermittently since it has many potential side effects if used all the time.

◆ It is sometimes difficult to obtain, so make sure your chemist keeps some in stock.

◆ *Enzyme inducing?*—No.

*Side effects*

◆ *Dose related*—ringing in the ears (tinnitus), tingling and unpleasant sensations in the limbs (paraesthesiae), and metabolic acidosis (the acid/alkali ratio in the blood is disturbed which can give rise to serious, widespread symptoms).

◆ *Hypersensitivity*—pathologically low white blood cell count, low blood platelet count, loss of production of new red cells (aplastic anaemia), rash, which includes Stevens–Johnson syndrome—rash, fever, and organ failure which can be fatal. Those hypersensitive to sulphonamide drugs should avoid it.

◆ *Chronic toxicity*—chronically low blood potassium (which can be serious) and metabolic acidosis (see above).

◆ *Does it affect the unborn baby?*—Yes in animal studies and therefore presumably in humans (no data). Since mainly used in women with premenstrual seizures better avoided in those actively trying to become pregnant.

◆ *Pregnancy*—if becoming pregnant whilst taking the drug is unavoidable take folic acid 5 milligrams by mouth every day from before you try to become pregnant and all the way through.

◆ *Breastfeeding*—effect on the baby totally unknown so best avoided except for the first few days.

## Clobazam

See entry in previous section on third-line drugs.

## Diazepam

The only use for this drug should be in an emergency to stop or ward off status or serial epilepsy by the intravenous route in hospital or by the rectal route (using a preparation such as Stesolid®) outside hospital.

If you are prone to status it may be worth teaching a few of your select friends who you are likely to be with (or your carer) how and when to administer rectal diazepam (and how much). The effective dose varies from person to person and should not be given more than once outside hospital (and, if it is successful in stopping your seizures—as it often is—it is still important to go to hospital as the effect may not last for very long with a clear written record as to how much was given and when). The rectal route may be embarrassing for you and raise practical and ethical issues for your friends and carers. The dose needed to stop your seizures without giving you too many side effects should be discussed with your doctor as it involves several different factors and may be a matter of trial and error.

An important side effect that you and your friends must be aware of is that too much rectal diazepam can seriously impair your breathing so you must sort out the dose carefully with your doctor. If you are going abroad into relatively undoctored parts and are going with a trusted companion and are liable to sudden bursts of seizures or prolonged ones it may be useful to take some rectal diazepam with you, and your colleague instructed as to when and how to use it. Use in labour will result in a very sedated baby, so if you are likely to have frequent seizures in labour their best management should be discussed with your specialist and a plan agreed and carefully noted. Blood levels of diazepam are not recorded clinically; it is not enzyme inducing.

## Rufinamide

This is a newly-launched drug specifically designed for children (and the first to be marketed specifically for them). It will be used, at least initially, for patients with the Lennox–Gastaut syndrome (a difficult-to-manage childhood epilepsy) but may of course, in time, expand its usefulness to other epilepsies; very much a case of 'watch this space'. Discuss its use and potential side effects with your medical advisor if you are offered it since it is a new drug.

# Obsolete drugs

## Ethosuximide

- ◆ An old drug, now little used, effective against primary generalized absences.
- ◆ Tonic clonic seizures often then supervene (since the drug cannot prevent them).

- It is very mildly enzyme inducing but not enough to significantly affect the blood levels of other anticonvulsant drugs.

- The side effects (including psychosis) can be severe and there is some (admittedly old) human data that the drug can damage the unborn baby.

- If you are still taking it (hopefully unlikely) arrange with your doctor to withdraw from it before you become pregnant—there are better and safer substitutes if you still need medication.

- If you find yourself pregnant whilst taking it hopefully you are taking folic acid 5 milligrams daily by mouth from before the pregnancy and throughout it.

- Arrange with your obstetrician for careful fetal scans to detect abnormalities during the pregnancy.

- Don't breastfeed for more than 4 or 5 days and arrange to withdraw from the drug when it is safe to do so before you become pregnant again.

- Blood levels are not routinely estimated and there is no evidence that they fall in pregnancy.

## Phenobarbital (old UK name phenobarbitone)

- Used for partial, secondarily generalized, and primary tonic clonic seizures.

- An old drug (almost the oldest anticonvulsant: bromide, no longer used, was the first).

- Still widely employed in less developed parts of the world because it is very cheap—a recent trial has shown it to be very effective in this setting.

- In the developed world now obsolete because of numerous side effects.

- In women should be avoided both in case of pregnancy and in the menopause.

- There is a quoted therapeutic blood level but there are doubts about its usefulness.

- *Enzyme inducing?*—Yes.

*Side effects*

- *Dose related*—sedation (can be severe even in low dose), unsteadiness, mental slowing.

- *Hypersensitivity*—rash.

- *Chronic toxicity*—megaloblastic anaemia (due to folic acid deficiency) and osteoporosis (bone thinning leading to risk of fractures due to interference with vitamin D absorption from the gut).

- *Does it affect the unborn baby?*—Fetal abnormality well described, so withdraw and substitute before becoming pregnant; if not take folic acid 5 milligrams orally from before the pregnancy starts and all the way through it.

◆ *Pregnancy*—in addition take vitamin K 10 milligrams daily by mouth from the 36th week until the end. No evidence that the dose has to be increased in pregnancy.

◆ *Breastfeeding*—for the first 4 or 5 days after birth certainly; thereafter be very cautious to avoid an overly sedated baby and it may be better not to.

## Phenytoin

◆ Used for partial seizures, secondary generalization, and primary tonic clonic.

◆ An old drug with many problems but still widely used (obsolete in the UK).

◆ Phenytoin is the one drug where blood level monitoring is essential.

◆ Having too high a blood level for too long can lead to irreversible damage.

◆ It is important to make sure that you stick to the same brand of phenytoin.

◆ There is a non-linear relationship between dose and blood level (unlike most drugs).

◆ A very small increase in the dose can push you beyond the therapeutic range.

◆ Blood level is misleading if taken with valproate: avoid this combination if at all possible.

◆ *Enzyme inducing?*—Yes.

### Side effects

◆ *Dose related*—unsteadiness, slurred speech, sickness, and double vision.

◆ *Hypersensitivity*—rash, pseudolymphoma (a condition mimicking cancer of the lymph glands), liver disease.

◆ *Chronic toxicity*—atrophy of the cerebellum (if high blood levels maintained for too long, leading to speech, walking, and co-ordination difficulties), megaloblastic anaemia (due to folic acid deficiency), osteoporosis (bone thinning due to failure to absorb vitamin D from the gut), overgrowth of the gums, undue hairiness, and coarsening of the skin of the face.

◆ *Does it affect the unborn baby?*—Yes, definite cleft lip and cleft palate, heart defects, microcephaly (small head), and failure of the nails and small bones in the hands to develop properly have all been described due in part, possibly, to a slow fetal heart rate caused by the drug. How much is preventable by high dose folic acid (one isolated report suggested that it might even increase abnormalities) is unknown. This does not mean that abnormality is inevitable; those few babies seen in the Birmingham Clinic born to mothers taking phenytoin were all quite normal and it may be that a lot of the abnormalities previously described occurred before blood level monitoring was introduced.

◆ *Pregnancy*—despite the one study suggesting a possible increase in abnormalities of the fetus in women taking high doses of folic acid with phenytoin we would advocate taking 5 milligrams of folic acid by mouth daily from before the pregnancy starts and all the way through plus 10 milligrams daily by mouth of vitamin K from the 36th week of the pregnancy until the end, although it would be better to have withdrawn from this drug and substituted, if necessary, before the pregnancy starts. Monthly monitoring of the blood level during pregnancy is essential with dose adjustments if required.

◆ *Breastfeeding*—not recommended by the manufacturers (but it is probably better to have some breastfeeding for the first 4 or 5 days to avoid abrupt withdrawal of the drug in the infant).

## Primidone

◆ A drug no longer recommended.

◆ Very similar to phenobarbital with all its drawbacks and should not be taken by women.

◆ If you are one of the 10,000 people in the UK still reported to be taking it then see your doctor for advice about withdrawal or substitution (in a study of chronic epilepsy carried out by Tim some years ago he was surprised by the number of patients taking both phenobarbital and primidone since they are, for all practical purposes, the same drug).

◆ Withdrawal should be slow.

◆ *Enzyme inducing?*—Yes.

## Vigabatrin

This drug, used against partial onset seizures with or without secondary generalization, had a reputation for causing a psychotic illness in some individuals (a bit like topiramate and probably for the same reason, too high an initial dose or too rapid an increase in dose) but, a few years after its introduction, it became apparent that in at least a third of the patients that took it a significant loss of peripheral vision occurred (the ability, when looking straight ahead, to see what is happening to the side). This loss is obviously potentially dangerous—it means, for instance, that driving a car would be too risky—and it appeared that it was probably irreversible once acquired (possibly not in children). As a result the drug is very little used: in the unlikely event that you are still taking the drug and were unaware of what you have just read then discuss with your medical advisor whether you should continue to take it and arrange for a specialist eye test including full perimetry (measurement of peripheral vision). The drug still has a small role (in skilled paediatricians' hands) in children with an otherwise difficult-to-treat and rare childhood epileptic condition (West syndrome).

*Enzyme inducing?*—No.

# Appendix 2

# Where else to find help and information

A specialist epilepsy clinic may have access to the information you need or will know where you can obtain it. Every country has at least one national epilepsy association; many have more than one (the British Isles, for instance, has separate Irish, Scottish, and Welsh organizations) and to print only a selection here would be invidious. Instead we will give you the address of the main UK body with a website address where you can find the address of every other organization in the world.

Epilepsy Action

New Anstey House

Gate Way Drive

Yeadon

Leeds LS19 7XY

For UK residents only: Freepost LS0995, Leeds, LS19 7YY

Telephone: 0113 210 8800

Freephone helpline: 0808 800 5050

International telephone: 0044 113 210 8800

Email: helpline@epilepsy.org.uk

Website: www.epilepsy.org.uk (links in searchbox)

Local organizations also exist in various large towns and districts often affiliated to national organizations. Most are helpful and supportive particularly for those of you starting out as a person with epilepsy or whose seizures do not rapidly come under control.

# Index